LEARNING IN PRACTICE FOR NURSING STUDENTS

LEARNING IN PRACTICE FOR NURSING STUDENTS

JESSICA MILLS

DARREN BRAND

 macmillan education   palgrave

First published 2018 by
PALGRAVE

Palgrave in the UK is an imprint of Macmillan Publishers Limited, registered in England, company number 785998, of 4 Crinan Street, London, N1 9XW.

Palgrave® and Macmillan® are registered trademarks in the United States, the United Kingdom, Europe and other countries.

ISBN 978–1–137–60454–5 paperback

This book is printed on paper suitable for recycling and made from fully managed and sustained forest sources. Logging, pulping and manufacturing processes are expected to conform to the environmental regulations of the country of origin.

A catalogue record for this book is available from the British Library.

A catalog record for this book is available from the Library of Congress.

Jessica Mills:
For my family
For Jareczka

Darren Brand:
For Maria, Jack & Paige

CONTENTS

LIST OF FIGURES

LIST OF TABLES

LIST OF BOXES

INTRODUCTION

Learning is about acquiring knowledge, skills and attitudes. Learning in practice for nursing students is no different. Over the duration of your course you will need to learn and successfully demonstrate the knowledge, skills and attitudes required for safe and effective practice as a registered nurse.

The premise of this book is to counter two fallacious statements made about student nurses' learning in practice. The first is a phrase heard commonly among nursing students that on any given placement: *'There is nothing to do and nothing to learn.'* Clearly, there will be unavoidable periods during your placement when there is less to do because of the restrictions of being a student. Yet the frequency with which students report this phenomenon suggests valuable opportunities are being missed to broaden and deepen your learning in practice.

The second erroneous statement is expressed by many nurses who suggest: *'You learn how to become a nurse once you are qualified.'* This misconception that your learning to become a nurse only really happens once you are registered undermines the value of learning in practice that you as a student dutifully and not without effort and cost undertake. To avoid regretting not making the most of your time as a student and your supernumerary status you need to maximise your learning in practice now.

The clinical learning environment should uniquely promote your learning by enabling you to apply what you learn at university to your practice and develop your critical thinking in the care of service users in real-time, real-life situations and interactions. It is not sufficient to just be in practice nor can it be assumed that you already have the requisite skills to be able to learn in practice. Despite your time in placement taking up half of the course there is limited guidance or indeed acknowledgement of the need for guidance about how to learn on your placement. At university, you will receive an abundance of advice about how to write essays and how to conduct literature searches, and you will be able to attend study skills sessions, workshops and tutorials. Surprisingly, there is not the equivalent volume of literature in existence that looks in detail at placement learning from the viewpoint of the student (the majority is from the perspective of the mentor and their role). Yet practice is an unfamiliar and often distracting learning environment compared to university lectures and seminars. This book is designed to directly support your learning and assessment in practice. It has six chapters which answer six questions, namely why you learn (Chapter 1), where you learn (Chapter 2), how you learn (Chapter 3), what you learn (Chapter 4), who you learn from (Chapter 5) and when you learn (Chapter 6).

Each chapter starts with learning outcomes that are achieved by working through the chapter and completing the associated activities. The activities have been designed to support, develop or target your learning. Some are more relevant to students who have as yet to attend practice but the majority are applicable to all students in all academic years and all nursing fields (adult, children's nursing, learning disabilities and mental health). Short vignettes from students are used to reinforce learning and also help you to identify with shared/common experiences. The information in the chapters is presented in a number of ways including figures, diagrams, tables and information boxes. At the end of each chapter there is a list of knowledge review questions covering key learning from the chapter with suggested answers provided in the relevant numbered appendices. A glossary is also provided and any words which are included in the glossary are written in bold. The book can be read cover to cover but it is anticipated that it will be more useful if used as a dip in and dip out text. Reviewing the index, learning outcomes and summaries for each chapter will assist you in identifying specific areas of information that you may want to research in more detail at different times throughout your course.

A brief synopsis of each chapter is provided. Chapter 1 – 'Why?' – provides a foundational understanding of why student nurses learn in practice by analysing the purposes and regulation of learning in practice and focusing on the individuals, communities and populations that you will learn to care for in practice. Chapter 2 – 'Where?' – defines the location of your learning. Your placement should be a clinical learning environment having fulfilled certain prerequisites and displayed positive attributes in order to enable you to achieve successful outcomes in your learning.

In Chapter 3 – 'How?' – you will develop an understanding of how you can learn best when you are in practice. You will explore your ability to learn and how to overcome challenges; you will identify your preferred learning style but also be encouraged to assimilate other styles to support your learning and accept responsibility for your learning. Chapter 4 – 'What?' – presents key learning needs for the knowledge, skills and attitudes required of a nurse. The emphasis in this chapter is on some of the more difficult to learn subjects such as decision making and care planning, rather than providing an exhaustive list of all the physical/technical skills you would need to be competent in as a nurse.

Chapter 5 – 'Who?' – examines who you learn from with advice on how you can get the best from your mentor. The ethics of learning on service users is studied along with the approach of interprofessional education and peer learning with your fellow students. In the final chapter, Chapter 6 – 'When?' – the time frames of when your learning happens are explored, that is, the time before, during and after your placement. Finally, the importance and process of assessment are explained as a means of confirming your achievement of learning.

Remember that what is unfamiliar to you and what you may be more information about is not universal. If your learning experience is different from your colleagues' you should not be put off from pursuing your own interests and learning needs. In your nursing education, you need to accept and adjust to the requirements of studying in higher education; you are considered to be an adult learner and, therefore, you are responsible for your own learning. As authors we hope that this book assists you in experiencing meaningful and transformative learning and as registered nurses we are confident that your learning in practice is vital to the development of the knowledge, skills and attitudes required of a nurse.

1

Why?

Learning outcomes

After reading and completing the activities in this chapter you will be able to:

➤ Explore the purpose of learning in practice.

➤ Identify the recipients of your nursing care.

➤ Explain the role of the Nursing and Midwifery Council in regulating nursing education in the UK.

As a student at university it should come as no surprise that you are here to learn. However, the course that you have chosen means that you are learning not just about a subject but how to become a professional. This is an important distinction as it means that your course is not just approved by the university but must also meet the requirements of the **Nursing and Midwifery Council** (NMC).

Shah's story (Children's nursing student)

'I had studied an English degree before I started my nursing degree and I found it really hard to adjust to the rules and regulations of the course. Simple things like signing a register and having to be in most days for lectures made me feel like I was back at school. Then my placements were even tougher. I had to get up crazy early and remember to iron my uniform. My other student friends who were not on my course were great but they did comment that it was much harder for me and they couldn't do it. But I know it was the right choice for me.'

The differences between nursing courses compared to most other courses at university are summarised in Table 1.1.

Table 1.1 Key differences of a nursing course

Course requirement	Details
Curriculum design and content	In addition to the curriculum set by the university, the course curriculum must adhere to the Nursing and Midwifery Council Standards.
Course regulation	In addition to approval by the university, the course must be approved by the Nursing and Midwifery Council.
Course review	In addition to periodic review of the course by the university, the course must be reviewed by the Nursing and Midwifery Council.
Course outcomes	In addition to achieving an academic qualification, on successful completion of the course the student will be eligible to register with the Nursing and Midwifery Council.
Service users	In addition to professional involvement, the course must have the involvement of service users in its design, delivery and student assessment.
Course components	50% of student attendance on the course is made up of time in the **clinical learning environment**.
Mandatory attendance	A student must complete a total of 4600 hours on the course in order to register with the Nursing and Midwifery Council. This total is made up of 2300 theory and 2300 practice hours.

These differences are likely to challenge your views and assumptions about what it means to be a student at university. Read the feedback students have given about their experience of being on a nursing course and then complete Activity 1.1 to help you reflect on your own thoughts and expectations of learning at university. This is a helpful exercise whether you have just started or you are in your final year.

Student nurse feedback on their nursing education

'My first few weeks at university were an exciting whirlwind.'
'She [final **sign-off mentor**] also encouraged me to think like a nurse by focusing on the whole patient not just the task.'

(Airey 2012)

'... contact with patients was a vital source of knowledge.'
'... even though [I was] actively searching for knowledge, [I felt] unsecure about [my own] ability.'

(Falk et al. 2016)

Activity 1.1 Reflecting on your learning

- What are/were your expectations of being a student at university?
- How closely do/did your expectations match your experiences?
- What do/did you enjoy learning?
- What concerns do/did you have about your learning?
- Do/did you know who to contact if you have/had difficulties with your learning?

This chapter answers the question why your nursing education comprises learning not just at university but also in practice. The chapter is divided into three sections. The first section explores the purpose of learning in practice; the second section presents the focus of learning in practice; and the final section details the regulation of your learning in practice.

The purpose of learning in practice

While the experience of learning is common to us all, you will have your own views and opinions as to the purpose of learning. This insight is most likely to have been formed during the period you spent in formal education, that is, at school and college. Many of you will have positive experiences of learning during this time; for others of you, however, your experience of learning may be associated with significant challenges and difficulties. These may relate to the process of your learning (i.e. how you learn) and/or the outcome of your learning (i.e. what you learn). While not wanting to dismiss your prior experiences, this section will affirm the purpose of learning in **higher education** specifically in relation to the time you spend in practice.

You will already be aware that even at school you did not just learn how to read, to write and to add up. You also learnt how to relate to your peers or those in authority, how to manage your time and how to communicate your thoughts, ideas and feelings through a range of media, for example writing, speaking, drawing even dance! It is unlikely that you were explicitly told that you would learn these skills and behaviours but having learnt them you are better equipped for living.

Schwarz (2016) expresses this as the 'joy of learning'. Whereby, in studying at university, the student gains a greater awareness of self, of others and of cultures, an appreciation of knowledge and learning, and becomes more receptive to diverse ideas and opinions. The hallmark of higher education is the development of advanced cognitive skills, that is, the ability to problem solve, to think critically, to be creative and to innovate. These elements can all be learnt during your time in practice.

Barbara's story (Children's nursing student)

'Wow, so I have such a respect for nurses. They have to think about so many different things plus more gets added to their 'to-do' list the longer they are on shift. I really like the problem solving. How can we make this child more comfortable? How do we keep this child from getting an infection when they are picking at their dressing? At one level it seems simple and we learn the right way to do things at university but putting it into practice definitely takes brain power.'

Education at university otherwise known as a **higher education institute** (HEI) is synonymous with **adult learning**. By assuming responsibility for your own learning, an adult will actively choose what and how they learn, whereas a child is more often a passive recipient of teaching (Knowles et al. 2012). Your readiness to learn will result from your own interest, curiosity and capabilities or an encounter in life which necessitates the need for you to understand something. Furthermore, as an adult you have a wealth of prior experiences and knowledge which act as a resource and a catalyst for your learning.

Nomsa's story (Mental Health nursing student)

'I would go back to my lecture notes and the books after most shifts because I realised I needed to figure out something about a drug or a disease or how to answer questions that service users would ask me but that I struggled to answer. Sometimes the lectures at university did not always match where I was at in practice but generally there was something I could go back to or I started to figure out where to look for the answers. It felt like I was really in control of my learning and how it was down to me.'

As a student on a nursing course you will definitely be considered as an adult learner. This may even have been explicitly written in the course literature. For example one of the aims of the course might be that you develop as an adult learner. The challenge for you is managing the course requirements in conjunction with the principles of adult learning, that is, exercising autonomy in what you learn and how you learn while achieving the professional standards required for registration. Consequently, the content of what you learn may not always align to your interests or be stimulated by your curiosity. Therefore, it is reasonable to expect a rationale for why certain content is included in (or excluded from) the **curriculum**. Similarly, as an adult learner you can ask if content absent from the curriculum could subsequently be incorporated.

André's story (Mental Health nursing student)

'When I got to uni, I was expecting some lectures on pharmacology. We were told about how to give drugs out and how important it was to get this right and know the side effects etc. But me and some other students were thinking 'shouldn't we know how drugs work too?' So we asked our course rep to bring this to the course lead and she added in some lectures. It was good to know that we could shape our learning.'

Your learning in practice is reliant on you being an adult learner – to identify your learning needs, to formulate your learning goals, to manage the resources and strategies needed to achieve these and to assess/evaluate the outcomes of your learning. This level of responsibility can seem somewhat daunting, but for most nursing students it is their time in practice which provides them with the greatest motivation to learn and succeed. The work by Müller and Louw (2004) clearly illustrates this. First, practice provides the student with the means to pursue their own interests and test out their capabilities. Secondly, it is only in practice that students experience a sense of satisfaction that occurs when they concentrate on and develop mastery of a task.[1]

The purpose of learning in practice will ideally strengthen your enjoyment of learning, foster your cognitive skills and form you as an adult learner. The fulfilment of this purpose is achieved through understanding the focus of learning in practice.

---

[1] 'Tasks' within the context of nursing practice include both clinical and non-clinical activities, for example communication, teamwork and so on.

The focus of learning in practice

Throughout your course, the focus of your learning in practice should be on those who receive your nursing care. This section will introduce the recipients of your nursing care as categorised by the NMC and present the current and projected healthcare needs of UK society.

The following descriptions of who will receive your nursing care and the standard of competency you need to achieve in this care are taken from the NMC Standards for Pre-registration Nursing Education (NMC 2010). The first two standards relate generically to all **nursing fields**. The subsequent standards apply to each separate nursing field, that is, adult, children's nursing, learning disabilities and mental health:

All nurses must work in partnership with **service users**, carers, families, groups, communities and organisations.

All nurses must be able to recognise and respond to the needs of all people who come into their care including babies, children and young people, pregnant and postnatal women, adults, people with physical health problems, mental health problems, people with physical disabilities, people with learning disabilities, older people, people with long-term conditions and those approaching the end of life.

Adult nurses must also be able to promote the rights, choices and wishes of all adults and, where appropriate, children and young people, paying particular attention to equality, diversity and the needs of an ageing population. They must be able to work in partnership to address people's needs in all healthcare settings.

Keith's story (Adult nursing student)

'To be honest I thought nursing was done in hospital. I had a vague idea of nurses on bikes going into people's homes but wasn't so interested. But these nurses really are on their own, they don't have a whole hospital to hand. It's not as random as paramedics doing their thing in a field but still nurses have to be a nurse in all sorts of places and at all times.'

Children's nurses must also be able to understand their role as an advocate for children, young people and their families, and work in partnership with them. They must deliver child and family-centred care; empower children and young people to express their views and preferences; and maintain and recognise their rights and best interests.

Annabel's story (Children's nursing student)

'It is fascinating learning about the anatomy and childhood development. I am always really excited about hearing the new treatments and advances there are in children's nursing. It is great to be in a profession that is dynamic and the work that I do directly benefits other people, children who will go on to live healthy lives as adults.'

Learning disabilities nurses must also be able to promote the individuality, independence, rights, choice and social inclusion of people with learning disabilities and highlight their strengths and abilities at all times while encouraging others do the same. They must facilitate the active participation of families and carers.

Jenny's story (Learning Disabilities nursing student)

'I did have quite a nurturing view of how to look after people with learning disabilities when I started and I soon came to realise that the people I was caring for could live independently or at least exercise some level of independence. I was learning not to just focus on the disabilities and health problems that someone had in their life but more on what they could do.'

Mental health nurses must also be able to work with people of all ages using values-based mental health frameworks. They must use different methods of engaging people, and work in a way that promotes positive relationships focused on social inclusion, human rights and recovery, that is, a person's ability to live a self-directed life, with or without symptoms, that they believe is meaningful and satisfying.

Farai's story (Mental Health nursing student)

'It is good that mental health nurses exist. I know all nurses should have knowledge of how things can go wrong physically and mentally for a person but the emphasis is different. It is about helping people make positive change and empowering them. It is hard seeing a change in someone's mental health and how it makes them incapable of looking after themselves, so knowing about human rights is important as we have to care for people even if they don't want it.'

It is important to recognise that your nursing care not only extends beyond the individual to the wider community but that your caring of others should also encompass **cultural sensitivity**. This is perhaps best summed up by the **World Health Organization** (WHO) in their vision statement from the 2010 Nursing and Midwifery Strategy which is reproduced in Box 1.1.

Box 1.1 World Health Organization Nursing and Midwifery Strategy 2010 – Vision statement

'Improved health outcomes for individuals, families and communities through the provision of competent, **culturally sensitive**, evidence-based nursing and midwifery services.'

Did you notice the opening sentence of this vision statement? The intention of your nursing care is that it should have a positive impact on people. This concept is embedded within the NMC Standards, which makes reference to empowering people to make helpful choices, to live self-directed lives and to address the needs of people in all healthcare settings. In 2015 the WHO Strategy on Nursing and Midwifery presented evidence of how the 2010 vision statement has been fulfilled by nurses throughout the world. Examples of health improvements achieved by nurses include:

➤ decreasing patient morbidity and mortality

➤ decreasing hospital readmissions, length of stay and healthcare acquired infections

➤ improving patient adherence with human immunodeficiency virus (HIV) and tuberculosis (TB) treatments

➤ reducing waiting times and the number of missed appointments through screening, triage and clinical intervention initiatives.

Implied within the NMC Standards (NMC 2010) is the understanding that the recipients of your care comprise not just those service users who are currently receiving health and social care but also all future recipients as well. The **International Council of Nurses** (ICN) spearheaded a global review of nursing (Bryant 2005). One of the core themes that emerged was:

Nursing students must learn how to be responsive to the needs of individuals and communities but also proactive in recognising trends and adapting to the prospective care needs of people and populations.

The following demographic information has been taken from the Office of National Statistics and presents an overview of the current and projected healthcare needs of people in the UK. Three key challenges are highlighted:

1. *Population growth in the UK:*
   The UK healthcare systems will have to plan for and accommodate a population increase which is predicted to grow by 7% reaching 68 million by 2022. For the ageing population the number of people over 85 in the UK is projected to increase from 1.4 million to 2.4 million by 2027 and to 3.6 million by 2037.

2. *Care for people with long-term conditions in the UK:*
   Of the current population, there are 150 million people living with **long-term conditions** accounting for 70% of the health spend. The current average cost for three conditions is approximately £8000 per year.

   By 2020, there will be a 30% increase in the number of people with three or more long-term conditions. Specific data on key long-term conditions:

   ➤ At the current trend 4 million adults will be diagnosed with diabetes by 2030.

   ➤ Chronic kidney disease is projected to rise to 4.2 million between 2011 and 2036 in adults.

   ➤ There is a projected increase by 40% over the next 12 years and by 156% in the next 38 years of adults with dementia.

   ➤ By 2035 it is predicted that 46% of men and 40% of women will be obese.

   ➤ The number of obese children doubles during the time children are at primary school.

   ➤ 1 in 7 children and young people are diagnosed with a long-term health condition or a disability.

   ➤ 1 in 10 children aged 5–16 years has a diagnosable mental health problem.

3. *Health inequalities for specific groups in the UK:*
   ➤ People with learning disabilities have significantly poorer health and increased age-adjusted mortality than other people (approximately one in 50 people have learning disabilities).

   ➤ People with severe and prolonged mental illness are at risk of dying on average 15–20 years earlier than other people.

➤ People with long-term physical illnesses suffer more complications if they also develop mental health problems, increasing the cost of care by an average of 45%.

➤ People living in the poorest areas will die on average 7 years earlier than those living in the richest areas.

➤ People from black and minority ethnic (BME) groups have poorer general health than the white British population.

➤ Depression, anxiety, alcohol and substance misuse are at least 1.5 times more common in lesbian gay bisexual transgendered and intersex (LGBTI) people, with lesbian and bisexual women at particular risk of alcohol abuse.

Above are some particularly concerning statistics that should provoke you to consider how, as a nurse, you can be involved in resolving/managing these issues. Work through Activity 1.2 to help you maintain inclusive practice for all recipients of your care.

Activity 1.2 Who receives your care?

Review this chapter section, then answer the following questions:

• How has your understanding of the recipients of your care been challenged or expanded?

• Who do you consider as a minority group within your nursing field?

• What health inequalities are people subject to in your nursing field?

• How could **unconscious bias** contribute to health inequalities?

• How will you resolve issues of health inequalities in your practice?

The focus of your learning in practice should be the recipient of your care. A recipient is identified by your field of nursing and encompasses the care provided at the level of both an individual and a population. This care should be delivered in a way that is culturally sensitive and that achieves positive health outcomes for all current and future recipients regardless of their ethnicity, age, gender or sexuality. By remaining focused on the recipients of your care, your learning in practice will be best directed towards acquiring the necessary knowledge, skills and attitudes. In order that the recipient of your care is safeguarded while you are a student, your learning in practice will be subject to the fulfilment of various mandatory provisions. The final section of this chapter will cover the regulation of your learning in practice.

The regulation of learning in practice

This section will outline the model of nursing education in the UK and its regulation, specifically in relation to learning in practice and the impact of higher education on UK nursing education.

The European Union (EU) published a directive in 2005 on healthcare education (Directive 2005/36/EC). Nursing education is referred to in article 31 of this directive. See Table 1.2 for a list of the mandatory requirements, related to the practice components of a nursing course, as set out in article 31. The directive establishes that nursing education should be provided by HEIs and regulated by a **Professional, Statutory and Regulatory Body** (PSRB). Over 140 HEIs across the UK are approved to deliver pre-registration nursing programmes. The NMC is the PSRB which regulates over 600,000 UK nurses and midwives. The NMC meets its PSRB condition of protecting the public by:

➢ setting and reviewing the required standards of nursing and midwifery education, conduct and performance

Table 1.2 The mandatory requirements of the practice components of a nursing course

Mandatory requirement	Practice component
Duration of learning in practice	2300 practice hours achieved over 3 years
Ratio of theory to practice hours	50% theory and 50% practice
Nature of learning in practice	The student learns as part of a team and in direct contact with a healthy or sick individual and/or community, to organise, dispense and evaluate the required nursing care
Assessment of learning in practice	The student is assessed on the basis of the knowledge, skills and attitudes which they have acquired
Role of the registered nurse	This learning will take place under the supervision of registered nursing staff
Types of practice	A range of practice in both hospital and community settings
Role of the PSRB	To approve the suitability of each practice area as a clinical learning environment using a mentor database and educational audits

> approving courses and programmes that provide nursing and midwifery education

> maintaining a register of practising nurses and midwives

> investigating any nurse or midwife who does not meet the required standards (see Activities 1.3 and 1.4).

Activity 1.3 The NMC Professional Register

Search for any nurses that you know on the NMC Professional Register: www.nmc.org.uk/

What information do you gain about the nurse from this search?

Activity 1.4 Attend a fitness to practice hearing

Consider attending a fitness to practice hearing during your course. The hearing will investigate the allegation(s) made against a nurse and impose the sanctions that the nurse must adhere to. For details of how to book: https://www.nmc.org.uk/concerns-nurses-midwives/hearings-and-outcomes/attending-a-hearing/

Alternatively review the transcripts of the fitness to practice hearings. What are your thoughts on:

• the types of allegations made against nurses?

• the sanctions imposed on nurses?

• the reputation of the nursing profession?

By acquiring the knowledge, skills and attitudes that meet the standards of education, conduct and performance required of a nurse, the NMC can reassure the public that once registered your practice is safe and effective. The relevant NMC standards of education, conduct and performance are:

> **Education** – *Standards for Pre-registration Nursing Education* (NMC 2010)

> **Conduct and performance** – *The Code: Professional Standards of Practice and Behaviour for Nurses and Midwives* (NMC 2015)

The details of each standard and how it relates to your learning in practice will now be explored.

Standards for Pre-registration Nursing Education (NMC 2010)

As a student on an NMC-approved pre-registration course you are required to meet these standards in full, in order to be eligible to join the professional register in a specific field of nursing: adult, children's nursing, learning disabilities or mental health. The standards have been formed into a **competency framework** which is set within four domains of nursing and with each domain there are related competencies. See Box 1.2 for the four domains and selected examples of the competencies. Complete Activity 1.5 to familiarise yourself with all the generic and field-specific competencies that must be assessed and achieved in practice.

Box 1.2 The four domains of nursing

1. Professional values

- promote health and well-being for individuals and communities
- maintain equality, diversity, inclusiveness and rights
- demonstrate compassion and dignity
- maintain autonomy, independence and self-care

2. Communication and interpersonal skills

- communicate effectively
- uphold an individual's identity and self-worth
- provide emotional support

3. Nursing practice and decision making

- develop critical thinking and decision making skills
- support physical health e.g. nutrition and hydration
- support mental health e.g. well-being, resilience
- respond to deterioration in health (physical and psychological)

4. Leadership, management and team working

- supervise, lead, manage and promote best practice
- manage risk
- manage information
- participate in effective teamwork

Activity 1.5 Competencies in nursing

Look up the generic and field-specific competencies for your nursing field: https://www.nmc.org.uk/globalassets/sitedocuments/standards/nmc-standards-for-pre-registration-nursing-education.pdf

Philippa's story (Learning Disabilities nursing student)

'Being a learning disabilities student nurse has meant I did not have to choose between adults or children in my nursing. I feel that in LD nursing you have to focus on the entire person and really understand their physical and mental health. It is great because you are involved in the client's whole life; it is not just about clinical or technical skills but also really being able to communicate. You learn how to do this with someone who has limited speech or understanding. When you get it right you can see the difference it makes; it's a real privilege.'

Michael's story (Adult nursing student)

'It was simple which field to choose but it has not been simple to learn. I don't regret my decision but I didn't really have any experience before. I was surprised at how much I was allowed to do, even on my first placement.'

The standards also refer to a range of essential skills for nurses. These skills support the achievement of the competencies by identifying a group of skills core to all nursing fields that should be learnt and assessed within practice. The skills are organised into five **essential skills clusters** (ESC):

1. care, compassion and communication
2. organisational aspects of care
3. infection prevention and control
4. nutrition and fluid management
5. medicines management

The NMC are clear that the ESC do not include all the skills and behaviours required of a registered nurse. This lack of uniformity can make establishing what you need to learn a somewhat nebulous task. Similarly, there are concerns regarding how applicable the, supposedly, essential skills are to all nursing fields. Use Activity 1.6 to test this out for yourself. Furthermore, the ESC could be criticised for being predominantly related to physical health with only limited reference to mental health for example.

Activity 1.6 How relevant are the ESC to your chosen field?

Look up the ESC: https://www.nmc.org.uk/globalassets/sitedocuments/standards/nmc-standards-for-pre-registration-nursing-education.pdf

- Why has this skill been included?
- How well does it align to your view of your field?
- What will/do you find easy to achieve?
- What will/do you find difficult to achieve?

Achievement of the NMC competencies and ESC are staggered throughout the course according to two **progression points** which separates the programme into three equal stages. The first progression point is normally at the end of year one and the second progression point is normally at the end of year two. The final stage is eligibility for entry to the professional register on successful completion of the course. Progression on the course is subject to you acquiring the minimum level of competence assigned to each progression point. The full criteria for each progression point are set out in 'Annexe 2 – Progression criteria' of the NMC Standards (NMC 2010). A summary of the progression points is available in Box 1.3.

Box 1.3 A summary of the NMC Progression criteria

Progression Point 1 requires the student to demonstrate the following:

- safety, safeguarding and protection of people of all ages, their carers and their families
- professional values, expected attitudes and the behaviours that must be shown towards people, their carers, their families, and others

▶

Progression Point 2 requires the student to maintain the competence achieved at Progression Point 1 and demonstrate the following:

- works more independently, with less direct supervision, in a safe and increasingly confident manner

- demonstrates potential to work autonomously, making the most of opportunities to extend knowledge, skills and practice

Entry to the register requires the student to maintain the competence achieved at Progression Points 1 and 2 and demonstrate the following:

- fulfilment of all generic and field-specific competences

The Code Professional Standards of Practice and Behaviour for Nurses and Midwives (NMC 2015)

The standards of conduct and performance for nurses are defined in *The Code: Professional Standards of Practice and Behaviour for Nurses and Midwives* (NMC 2015) referred to hereafter as The Code. While registered nurses must adhere to The Code, you will also be expected to observe the same required practices and behaviours as a student. Over the period of your nursing education you will need to develop your understanding and demonstration of The Code in your practice. Use Activity 1.7 to help you in this process.

Activity 1.7 Developing your nursing practice and behaviour according to The Code

Look up The Code

https://www.nmc.org.uk/globalassets/sitedocuments/nmc-publications/nmc-code.pdf

- Read through The Code

- What are the four areas in The Code?

- What aspects of The Code match your expectations of nurses' practice and behaviour?

- What aspects of The Code are new to you?

- What does The Code say about nurses' practice and behaviour towards students?

- How would you evidence in your own practice and behaviour that you are adhering to The Code?

Your nursing programme

Your nursing programme, in order to meet the NMC Standards, must provide you with learning opportunities at university and in practice. Both of these areas will equally contribute to your progression on the course and development as a nurse. Therefore, one area cannot be deemed of greater or lesser value than the other. Principally, this is because one area will naturally reinforce learning in the other. For example, your assessments may require you to reflect on a clinical experience or you may need to research and critique the evidence base for a particular nursing skill when you are on placement. Activity 1.8 will help you look at the structure of your course in relation to your learning in practice and determine how well your course enables you to meet the required NMC Standards while you are in practice.

Activity 1.8 Your nursing course – a review

- How is your learning in practice scheduled?
    - o Are you allocated to a placement pathway?
    - o How are you guaranteed a range of placements?
    - o Are you able to choose your own placements?
- How is your learning in practice utilised?
    - o Which, if any, modules make reference to your learning in practice?
    - o Is your learning in practice supported by simulation?
    - o What guidance do you receive to prepare for your placements?
    - o What support is available to you during your placements?
    - o How is your learning in practice assessed/evaluated?

Many of the learning experiences that you have in practice will be similar to those you encounter at university, for example seminars, lectures and **simulation**. You will also have different learning experiences in the practice setting that either cannot be easily taught at university or are achievable only in practice. Examples of these types of learning experiences include:

Learning about learning

➤ relate theory directly to practice

➤ develop skills of self-directed study

> develop skills of **reflection** and self-awareness

> prepare for and achieve practice-based assessments.

Learning about the nursing profession and other professions

> develop professional role identity

> establish values and beliefs about nursing

> socialisation into the profession

> work within the context of interprofessional and interagency working

> function within teams and organisations

> transition from student to registered nurse.

Learning about nursing care

> emersion within the clinical environment

> integration and engagement with clinical experiences

> recognise the varying responsibilities of the nurse according to the clinical setting

> become capable and skilled in the delivery of care (clinical and non-clinical skills)

> acquire the knowledge and attitudes of nurses such as language, behaviours, clinical decision making and so on.

Olivia's story (Adult nursing student)

'I was really enjoying the lectures, most of the time, but it just made me more desperate to get out in practice and have a go. I was really pleased that what I had heard about in university I actually saw. But I also realised that there is a big difference. The focus on you as a student is different. I liked the one-to-one which you don't really get at uni but sometimes it was easier to ask if I didn't understand something in a lecture.'

Julian's story (Mental Health nursing student)

'I kind of needed time to unpack my learning from practice. It is a faster pace of learning and not as logical or as planned. For a lecture you get the notes before to

▶

◀

prepare and you know what is coming up. But when you are in practice you are learning lots but it is not so obvious or in a way you expect. This took me some time to figure out and I realised I had to use the assessment book and the modules I was studying to narrow and focus my learning. I then didn't feel like I was missing out, I was more in control of my learning. If the course is planned right you will cover everything and you just have to know it will happen and make the most of it when it does.'

Learning in practice – regulations

In fulfilment of the EU Directive you are required to achieve 2300 hours in direct contact with **service users**. This translates to 50% of the minimum duration of your course being allocated to time in practice. This mandatory time in practice, facilitated by your programme providers, should be both effective and integral to the programme to enable you to achieve competence as a nurse. You should have access to a range of placements, including community, hospital, intermediate care, private and third-sector settings with experiences that cover the whole 24 hours, 7 days a week time period.

Specific provisions for your practice learning include:

➤ A period of at least four weeks of continuous practice learning towards the end of the first year and again at the end of year two.

➤ A period of at least 12 weeks of practice learning at the end of the programme in year three, to enable the **sign-off mentor** to make a judgement regarding achievement of the required standards of competence for entry to the NMC register.

➤ If you do not achieve your practice hours, and this can be for several reasons – such as sickness, expected and unexpected absences, incomplete attendance records – your completion of the course may be delayed, and you may be required to complete additional practice hours to meet the 2300 hours minimum.

➤ You must be allocated a **mentor** who will supervise you in practice.

➤ You must retain your **supernumerary** status when in practice.

Supernumerary status

Programme providers must ensure that students are **supernumerary** during all practice learning opportunities. Having supernumerary status means that as a student you will not, as part of your course, be contracted by any person or body to provide nursing care. The placements have a contractual obligation to support your learning and protect your supernumerary status. According to Smoker (2010) this is a fundamental principle of nursing education as it gives *you* the student the freedom and time to learn. Your supernumerary status supports your presence in practice and establishes the practice area for you and your mentor as a **clinical learning environment** (CLE). See Chapter 2 – 'Where?' – for more information on this.

Jessica's story (Adult nurse)

'I did not make the most of being a student in practice. When I look back now I wish I had asked more questions and really made the time to get my head round things. It is much more awkward 5 years on as a registered nurse to not know things than it ever was as a student.'

'I can see that my experience as a registered nurse has helped me to develop but I still think I could have made it easier on me by using the excuse of being a student to go anywhere and ask anything to build up my knowledge and skills when I had the time. Which I definitely don't have now!'

During your course you may have times on placement when your supernumerary status is undermined or threatened and as a result you may feel like you are 'just a pair of hands'. For example, on a busy ward, rather than working with your mentor, you are told to work with the healthcare assistant or support worker, with the intention that you contribute to the completion of their role such as assisting people with toileting, washing and dressing, mobilising, eating and drinking, monitoring, cleaning, stock checks and so on. Alternatively, you may view your supernumerary status as too restrictive: rather than there being too much to do there is too little as you encounter the limitations of what a student can do while under supervision. In either eventuality you are faced with choices about your learning – Do you develop the confidence to say no? Do you raise concerns about the loss of your supernumerary status? Do you question the learning situation? Or do you think how you can turn each situation into a learning opportunity?

Understandably, you will encounter periods throughout your nursing education when you have limited knowledge or when you struggle to develop skills or demonstrate the required behaviours. You may also experience relief when your mentor steps in and takes over or you may be glad that you are not yet registered as you comprehend the gap between where you are now and where you need to be as a registered nurse. However, your supernumerary status should never mean that you introduce yourself as being 'only' or 'just' a student nurse. The risk of excusing your presence in practice and your need to learn while as a student is that this could translate to when you are registered and you then start to say 'I am only a nurse'. The nursing profession should be made up of people who are proud to be a member of their profession and have a self-awareness of their current capabilities and the importance of **continuous professional development**.

Impact of higher education on nursing education

The most significant change in nursing education in recent years is the NMC requirement for degree-only entry to the professional register from 2011 onwards. At some point during your course you may ask yourself the question: 'Do I really need a degree to be a nurse?' This may be in response to public or media opinion, to nurses who criticise the value of a degree in comparison to their own nursing education or simply when you are faced with the task of writing your dissertation. The answer as to whether nurses need to have a degree is a resounding yes!

Higher academic achievement at the pre-registration stage arguably equips nurses earlier with the required skills for the profession (Buerhaus et al. 2016). For example, research over the last decade repeatedly demonstrates improved patient outcomes, including reduced mortality rates (i.e. how many people die), with higher employment levels of nurses holding a degree (Clark et al. 2015; Matthias 2015). Smoker (2010) identifies that the purpose of learning at university, that is, developing skills in problem solving, critical thinking and so on, are absolutely required by the registered nurse who will need to think through practice issues, to take ideas forward, to promote change in practice and to advance the nursing profession.

The latest review of nursing education was published in the *Shape of Caring Review: Raising the Bar* (Willis 2015). The review aimed to ensure consistent high-quality education to support high-quality care. The review makes specific recommendations for the practice-based component of nursing education in that it should be delivered and assessed against clear standards and provided within a supportive infrastructure. This approach acknowledges that it is not sufficient for you to just attend practice but rather the time you spend in practice needs to be quality assured, planned and directed in order for effective learning to occur. This will remain part of the NMC's quality assurance process when they produce new pre-registration nursing education standards in the next year.

Summary

This chapter has reviewed the purpose, focus and regulation of your learning in practice. The purpose is to enable you to develop the necessary cognitive skills (such as critical thinking and problem solving) within the real-time situations that you will only encounter on placement. Additionally, as an adult learner your experiences in practice will support your learning to become more self-directed. Finally the purpose of practice is to provide you with the satisfaction of testing out your capabilities and of developing an interest in your own learning.

The focus of your learning should be on the recipients of your nursing care. The range of recipients (from the individual to populations) according to each nursing field has been summarised. The importance of caring in a culturally sensitive way and improving the health outcomes of all was also addressed. Further, by acknowledging the current and future healthcare needs in the UK you will be able to direct your learning in practice to respond to changing needs, developments, priorities and expectations in the healthcare of individuals and communities.

The regulation of your practice ensures that you uphold the reputation of the profession and achieve safe and effective practice. The model and regulation of nursing education in the UK was presented with specific reference to learning in practice such as the mandatory practice hours, the competencies to be achieved in practice and the importance of your supernumerary status. The impact of higher education on nursing education was also explored.

As a nurse you will be required to practise autonomously: using the best available evidence, skilfully using technology and maintaining the person at the centre of your nursing care. You must be able to lead, delegate, supervise and challenge other nurses and healthcare staff. You will be required to develop practice and advance the nursing profession. In order for this to happen you must learn in practice the required knowledge, skills and attitudes to comprehensively take on the role and the responsibilities of a registered nurse.

Knowledge review

See Appendix 1 to compare your answers.

1. What are the benefits to the learner of completing higher education?

2. What is an appropriate term to describe a key attribute of an adult learner?

3. What document must all nursing programmes in the UK adhere to?

4. How many theory and practice hours comprise a UK nursing course?

5. What are some of the unique elements/advantages of learning in practice?

Further reading and resources

British Library Social Welfare Portal: Report on minority groups: https://www.bl.uk/social-welfare

Chief Nursing Officer bulletin: https://www.england.nhs.uk/tag/chief-nursing-officer/

Department of Health, Social Services and Public Safety: https://www.dhsspsni.gov.uk/

International Council of Nurses: http://www.icn.ch/

NHS England: https://www.england.nhs.uk/

> Health Education England: https://hee.nhs.uk/

NHS Northern Ireland: http://online.hscni.net/

> Northern Ireland Practice and Education Council for Nursing and Midwifery: http://www.nipec.hscni.net/

NHS Scotland: http://www.healthscotland.com/

> NHS Education for Scotland: http://www.nes.scot.nhs.uk/

NHS Wales: http://www.wales.nhs.uk/

> Workforce, Education and Development Services: http://www.weds.wales.nhs.uk/home

Nursing and Midwifery Council: https://www.nmc.org.uk/

Office of National Statistics: https://www.ons.gov.uk/

World Health Organization: http://www.who.int/en/

2

Where?

Learning outcomes

After reading and completing the activities in this chapter you will be able to:

> Define the **clinical learning environment** (CLE).

> Recognise the prerequisites of the CLE.

> Explore the attributes of the CLE.

> Examine the outcomes of the CLE.

This chapter starts with an activity (see Activity 2.1) to help you determine what you like or dislike about practice. As you will spend the equivalent of 50% of your course time in practice, it would make sense that you are able to enjoy or at least appreciate being in practice. Understandably, your preferences and even your prejudices about practice will influence your learning. It is, therefore, helpful at an early stage to manage or challenge your expectations and assumptions and to remain open-minded to each new practice experience that you enter.

Your practice experiences will occur within specific clinical areas often referred to as **placements**. You will experience a range of placements in order to ensure that you meet the **Nursing and Midwifery Council** (NMC) requirement of 2300 practice hours (this total can include up to 300 **simulation** hours). A common configuration of placements is a system of block learning, whereby students will attend either a block of time at university or a block of time on placement. Generally, there will be an equal number of university and practice blocks but the hours you attend at university will often be fewer in comparison to the hours you spend on placement. The additional theory hours will be comprised of independent study.

Activity 2.1 What do you like or dislike about being in practice?

Think about where you (would) like to go in practice and list the reasons for this.

- Is it because of convenience, familiarity, good reputation (according to whom?)?
- Is it because of what you may learn, experience?
- Is it because of preference?
- Is it because of the people (staff, students, service users)?
- Is it because of other commitments (academic, personal, health)?

Now think about where you do not (would not) like to go in practice and list the reasons for this.

- Is it because of inconvenience, unfamiliarity, poor reputation (according to whom?)?
- Is it because of what you may not learn, experience?
- Is it because of no preference?
- Is it because of the people (staff, students, service users)?
- Is it because of other commitments (academic, personal, health)?

Review your answers and think what needs to change to make you consider every practice area as somewhere you (would) like to go to.

Shah's story (Children's nursing student)

'Most of my placements so far have been great; and I am starting to know what I like and don't like. I had an idea what I might prefer before I started but it is often so different once you are in the clinical area and your role as a student is also not the same as if you were a staff member so that also changes your opinion about a placement.'

Alternative programme structures may include time each week in university and on placement, for example you have one or more days at university and one or more days in practice in the same week. Or you may experience a combination of block learning and integrated university and practice time. The configuration of your time in practice has been designed to support your learning. Try Activity 2.2 to help you think more about the purpose of attending a placement.

Activity 2.2 What do you think the purpose of a placement is?

Is it just to ensure you achieve the 2300 practice hours?

What else could it be about?

At an organisational level, the placement simply refers to the clinical area that a student has been allocated to attend. However, your attendance on placement is not just about clocking up the required hours; rather it is (or should be) about your learning to become a nurse. Therefore a more comprehensive term used throughout this book and in the related literature refers to the placement as the **clinical learning environment** (CLE). The CLE is the place where you as a student will learn to apply your knowledge, skills and attitudes in a real-time setting in order to prepare you for professional practice as a nurse. Essentially, the CLE facilitates what cannot be learnt elsewhere on the course even with the most sophisticated high-fidelity simulation and the most engaging clinically credible lecturers. Participation in the CLE is therefore integral to your course and your development as a nurse.

Nomsa's story (Mental Health nursing student)

'From being in placement I have learnt that nurses have to lead and therefore I need to develop these skills. Seeing what nurses actually do day to day means I have had to focus on skills much earlier than I thought I would. So the leadership skills for example I thought would only come once I was registered and wanting to become a ward sister, but nurses lead from day one.'

Barbara's story (Children's nursing student)

'It soon dawned on me when I was in practice the knowledge I needed to have. That 'bunny in headlight' feeling of not knowing definitely felt more real and immediate when on placement compared to university. In a lecture if I do not know the answer or do not understand something there is time to find out or we get the answer anyway.'

Jenny's story (Learning Disabilities nursing student)

'As I had worked as a support worker I had a good idea of what nurses needed to know and do. The bit that I had no clue about and I now realise is just as important is how to manage the competing demands, prioritising the care needs of different clients. Getting all the jobs done is like a balancing act and this is hard but really important to learn.'

Keith's story (Adult nursing student)

'For me the most important skill I am learning is how to apply what I have learnt. It almost does not matter where I learnt it; at university, on placement or in the library what has to happen when I am in practice is figuring out how to use this knowledge or skill or way of being with a patient. Nothing comes in a neat package with clear instructions to make use of straight away.'

In comparison with the university classroom, the CLE is a more dynamic and socially complex setting. As a result, you will have to overcome distractions and accept that your learning may be more disjointed or ad hoc. This, coupled with the sense of unfamiliarity and the feeling of repeatedly starting over with each new placement, can mean that your learning in practice is far less conducive. By exploring the prerequisites, the attributes and the outcomes of the model CLE, this chapter will help you successfully manage and negotiate your learning in practice.

The prerequisites of the CLE

There are two prerequisites that must be met in order for a placement to be considered a suitable CLE for a student nurse: it must be safe and supportive for students; and it must adhere to the quality assurance standards. This section will define these prerequisites and give you advice on how to manage difficulties if or when these prerequisites are not met.

Safe and supportive CLEs

Your safety and that of the **service user** is of paramount importance. Therefore, prior to attending your first placement, you should receive training in basic life support, moving and handling, health and safety, fire, safeguarding and information governance. You will be required to repeat some of these elements annually. Depending on the type of CLE you may also be required to attend additional training such as lone worker (community), breakaway training or first aid.

You should be aware of the process for raising and escalating concerns and the support available for you in the event of reporting a concern. Within each CLE that you attend you should also be given an induction to go through elements such as risk assessment, incident reporting and emergency procedures. Finally, service users and carers should be informed that student nurses may be involved in their care and that they have the right to decline the care of a student.

Difficulties in relation to safe and supportive CLEs

The most obvious difficulty or risk is exposing service users to unsafe care by students. As a novice rather than an expert you are vulnerable to making inadvertent mistakes resulting from acts of commission or omission, that is, you did something when you should not (commission) or you did not do something when you should (omission). **The Code** (NMC 2015) is clear that you should work within your competence but that if you make a mistake that you should be open and candid about this.

Julian's story (Mental Health nursing student)

'I have had a few sleepless nights during my course where I have woken up having forgotten to do something in the day on my placement. My mentors were fine about it but it stayed with me for quite a while and made me realise how important it is to be under supervision and keep checking-in with my mentor.'

The supervision you receive from your **mentor** will be a safeguard against you making mistakes. You will likely work alongside your mentor observing their practice first before you are allowed to undertake the same practice yourself. Developing self-awareness of your own competence will also enable you to monitor your progress and identify areas where you may require more direct supervision and/or further learning and assessment of your knowledge, skills and attitudes. In the event that you are involved in or witness an incident/near miss you are required to report this (see Activity 2.3).

**Activity 2.3 What should you do in the event of an incident/
near miss?**

As part of your induction to each placement you should be informed of the incident
reporting procedure. What are the key aspects of this procedure that you remember?

On your next placement review the last 3–6 months' incidents/near misses:

- What are the types of incident/near miss?
- Can you spot any trends?
- What has changed as a result of the incident/near miss?

Review Section 14 of The Code (NMC 2015)

A second difficulty that you may experience in the CLE is one of feeling exposed. There will be no lecture hall to hide in, unlike being at university; you will invariably be on your own in placement. This means it is your knowledge, skills and attitudes and not that of your colleagues that will be under scrutiny. Again the role of the mentor is to support and guide you. Therefore, if you feel worried or anxious about any aspect of your placement, do share these concerns with your mentor. It is perfectly normal to feel nervous, but you need to ensure that these nerves do not impact upon your ability to learn. See Chapter 3 – 'How?' – for more information on the range of people available to support you in practice and how to build up your resilience and manage your anxiety.

The final difficulty that you may encounter is one of witnessing poor practice. The overwhelming majority of nurses and other healthcare professionals intend to deliver safe and effective care. On occasions, however, there may be factors that inhibit or restrict a nurse's ability to deliver the highest standard of care possible – but there is a distinct difference between this and poor practice. You will learn about the ethical and legal requirements of being a nurse and your responsibility to adhere to The Code. You will be aware that you have a duty under The Code to report any concerns relating to practice that you have observed. If you feel unable to approach your mentor or another colleague to report it, do use the alternative reporting mechanism available within the university. Either way, the university will support you in reporting your concerns.

Speaking up is something that may trouble you, and for the majority of us it does not come easily. You may have the following questions: What if I am wrong? Do I really understand what I am seeing? Will others believe what I am saying? These reservations are natural, but they should not put you off from raising concerns. Complete Activity 2.4 to ensure you are fully aware of how to report practice concerns.

Activity 2.4 Reporting concerns

In the event that you witness or are aware of practice that does not uphold the law and professional standards do you know what to do next?

Spend some time finding out if your course has a policy on reporting or making concerns known? Who will you contact? Who will support you in the process? What happens when you report a concern?

Quality assurance of the CLE

An educational audit of each CLE should be completed every two years in partnership with practice and university staff and should review the CLE across the following areas:

➢ the maximum capacity of students

➢ the accuracy of the database of suitably registered mentors, sign-off mentors and practice teachers

➢ the appropriateness of the teaching and learning strategies offered

➢ the resourcing and evaluation of the teaching and learning strategies

➢ the reliability and validity of the practice assessments that are conducted

➢ the feedback mechanisms to monitor individual student progression between practice and university

➢ the preservation of a student's supernumerary status

➢ the placement profile should be reviewed regularly and updated accordingly to take account of any changes to service provision.

Difficulties in relation to the quality assurance of CLEs

The quality assurance difficulty most commonly reported by students is the provision of mentors and their ability to mentor. Chapter 5 – 'Who?' – has more detail on the role of the mentor as you should experience it in practice; however, the following are examples of some typical issues that you may experience with suggested solutions.

The mentor's inability to balance delivering patient care with the responsibilities of supervising a student nurse

This could be due to a change in the service user's condition, a shortage of staff within the department or a lack of experience on the part of the mentor. You will need to become accustomed to such situations, and develop your own strategies to ensure that your learning can continue. To help you manage this, remember that you are required to spend only 40% of your placement time under direct or indirect supervision with your mentor. Therefore, you should fully expect for the majority of your placement to work alongside other staff.

The mentor not knowing what you to do with you

This could be due to a lack of clear expectations on the part of the mentor and explicit learning needs on the part of the student. By ensuring that you meet with your mentor early in your placement, you can devise a mutually agreed **learning contract** that will set out what you intend to achieve, and the expectations of the mentor and the wider clinical team. Your mentor has a facilitative role, therefore as an **adult learner** you will be expected to be proactive and responsible for your own learning. Should you find yourself in the position of continually observing rather than participating in practice, you should initially approach your mentor to establish the reason why you are only observing. Generally, there should be no reason why you cannot fully immerse yourself in the activity of the placement. Exceptions to this would be:

➤ your level of competence

➤ policy which precludes a student nurse participating in specific care activities

➤ a service user who refuses to consent to care given by a student nurse.

If the issue persists, you would need to consider approaching either the nurse in charge or the university to seek a resolution.

The mentor not completing the Assessment of Practice document

Mentors are aware that your time in practice should be evidenced and documented. Therefore, not completing the document may be due to the mentor's lack of familiarity and/or time for its completion. Students are often concerned that they are pestering their mentor to get the document filled in; however, you would be supported by staff within practice and at university if you have to raise this as a concern. Being really familiar with the document yourself, for example knowing which sections are mandatory and optional (if any), will help you guide your mentor. Chapter 3 – 'How?' – provides full information on the Assessment of Practice document and its completion.

A further difficulty related to the quality assurance of the CLE is the appropriateness of the teaching offered to you during the placement. In order to establish your learning contract and manage your learning experiences it is important that the nature of the placement – what you will experience/encounter – is made known to you. Unlike your time in university, the nature of learning in the CLE is unpredictable and therefore students are at risk of not being provided with adequate and fair opportunities to learn and be assessed. Each placement setting should have a **placement profile** which will give you key information about the placement including staff contact details, a description of the healthcare activities undertaken in the clinical area and the available learning opportunities. The placement may also have a welcome pack or education resource with journal articles and items of interest that directly relate to the work of that area. You would also be encouraged to complete an evaluation at the end of the placement to give feedback on your learning experience in the CLE.

The final difficulty you may encounter is preserving your supernumerary status while on placement. This can be especially difficult if you have previous healthcare experience as you may be more prone to offer service provision at the expense of participating in learning opportunities. Likewise, the immediacy of service users' needs can be hard to overlook. Although you would not be expected to ignore service users, it is important that while in practice you remain a learner and not an unofficial employee. Typical periods when your supernumerary status may be at risk are during the winter months when there may be more staff sickness compounded by increased admissions and in the summer months when there may be more staff taking holidays. However, you should have a low threshold for flagging this as it will compromise your learning. Initially speak with your mentor and/or the nurse in charge. You should also contact the university and explain the situation. Observing how the supernumerary status of a student is achieved and maintained in different placements is also a helpful exercise as you can introduce solutions to new CLEs from your prior experiences.

Precious's story (Adult nursing student)

'Our practice books have a statement about being supernumerary and we were told by university to report any issues asap. I spoke with my personal tutor about this and she made me see that by using students to support the care of patients means the shortfall in care is never flagged up. Plus I do not have the same status or rights as an employee and it rarely involves working alongside my mentor so I am neglecting the reason to be there in the first place.'

The attributes of the CLE

Having established the necessary prerequisites of the CLE, each CLE should also display key qualities that ensure it is a positive environment for learning. The ideal attributes of a CLE encompass not only the different types of placement but also the availability of a range of learning opportunities and an organisational culture that supports and promotes learning in practice.

Types of placement

The NMC will have approved the quality and range of placements available to you on your course. The expectation is that you will experience a diverse range of healthcare within hospital and community settings from the **National Health Service** (NHS), private, voluntary and independent (PVI) sectors. See Table 2.1 for examples of placements according to sector. Balanced against this requirement will be the specifications of your programme, the availability of placements and the capacity of placements to accommodate students. While a considerable amount of effort goes into planning and managing the allocation of your placements, it is unrealistic to expect that each of your placements will directly align to where you are at on the course. The only time this may occur purposefully is in the event of your course offering you a choice of placement or on your final placement which will have been organised to enable you to complete specific competencies and skills.

Your placements will take place in a wide range of clinical settings, from acute wards, clinics, through to community services and people's own homes. For the majority of students, most of your placements are likely to be within the NHS although you should expect to gain

Table 2.1   Placements according to healthcare sector

Healthcare sector	Placement type
NHS	Personal care service Community nursing General practice Health visitor Paramedic/ambulance service Mobile clinic Minor injury unit Walk-in centre Assisted living Residential care Nursing home Hospital Rehabilitation Hospice
Private	Personal care service Community nursing Private clinic Assisted living Residential care Nursing home Hospital Rehabilitation Hospice
Voluntary	Community day centre/support group Charity day centre/support group Hospice
Independent	School Assisted living Residential care Nursing home

experience in the PVI sector as well. The NHS is a large and very complex organisation that is constantly evolving and reconfiguring to meet the needs of the public it serves. You only have to read a newspaper, or watch the news on television, to understand that the NHS is under significant pressure, supporting a growing population that is living longer and expecting free access to treatments and technologies that have a considerable cost associated with them. You will be able to learn how the service is managed at a local, regional and national level, what the experience is like for staff and servicer users alike, the impact of limited resources on service provision and how innovation and research can influence operational and strategic change.

There is an outmoded view of nursing education that negates certain care environments such as nursing homes as of little value to student learning but this shows a limited view of nursing and diminishes the professional role of the nurse as an autonomous, independent professional (Brown 2013). A sign that your course is getting your placement provision right is if you experience a variety of health and social care-related placements so that you are equally prepared for work in a hospital or the community.

> ### Philippa's story (Learning Disabilities nursing student)
>
> 'I am enjoying the different placements, although getting used to each new placement can be tricky but it is getting easier as I am figuring out how to prepare better for each new one.'

Learning opportunities

Each placement can and should offer you a wealth of teaching and learning opportunities. The availability of these opportunities depends on the facilitation skills of the mentor, sufficient variation in the care activities and the level of student engagement in their learning (Flott and Linden 2016). Refer to Chapter 3 – 'How?' – for details of how to learn in practice and Chapter 4 – 'What?' – for specific examples of what can be learnt in different placement settings. Part of the process of managing your learning while on placement is to think creatively about where your learning can happen. By way of a general distinction, student nurses identify they learn more about a holistic approach to care and autonomous nursing practice within the community as opposed to the acute setting (Krol et al. 2016). You may also be able to supplement placement learning by participating in sessions from a rolling teaching programme, joining staff on an in-house study day or attending conferences.

A commonly utilised method to maximise where your learning can happen is the **hub and spoke model**. In this model each individual placement acts as 'the hub' which then has conjoined 'spoke' experiences of varying number (see Figure 2.1). Think of the hub as your base (with the usual pattern of a named mentor who supervises your practice and facilitates your learning) from which you will plan and complete additional learning as spokes. The duration of the spoke experiences will vary from a couple of hours through to a number of days. The spoke may involve attending a different practice setting and/or working alongside another practitioner (nursing, medical, allied health, social care,

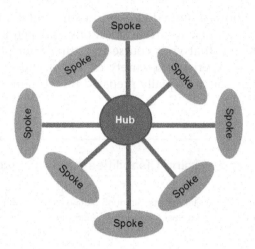

Figure 2.1 Hub and spoke model

education and so on). The spokes should be arranged in conjunction with your mentor who can then approve the suitability and feasibility of the experience. An alternative configuration of the model is having a dedicated hub placement to which you return at varying times throughout the three years and the spoke experiences are secondary placements to supplement the learning gained within the hub placement.

The benefit of this model is the hub placement promotes and enhances your sense of belongingness which has been identified as a key determinant of learning (Falk et al. 2016). The spokes will enable you to shape your individual learning experiences while at the same time fostering professional collaboration with your mentor when you are arranging the spokes and with other health and social care professionals when you attend the spokes. Table 2.2 has examples of the different types of spokes available with a rationale.

Organisational culture

The final attribute of the CLE is its organisational culture. Culture encompasses the written and unwritten rules and social mores of the organisation that determines staff socialisation, establishes the practice ethos and governs the working patterns of staff (Muls et al. 2015). Within this context, the organisational culture will influence the value placed on learning and whether the practice setting can even be considered a CLE. As a student you will need to gauge the effect of the culture

Table 2.2 Examples of spoke experiences with rationales

Type of spoke	Examples	Rationale
Arrange regular visits	• Attend a weekly outpatient clinic • Arrange repeated visits to a family/service user over an extended period of time	• Avoid one-off interest visits • Enhance an understanding of person-centred care and the service user experience/perspective • Gain an appreciation of service provision • Gain exposure to a wider range of CLEs
Follow a service user journey	• Attend a pre-assessment clinic, operating theatre department and post-surgery outpatients • Attend a day centre/other care activities that the service user participates in	• Enhance an understanding of person-centred care and the service user experience/perspective • Gain an appreciation of service provision • Gain exposure to a wider range of CLEs
Arrange specialist experiences related to the practice area	• Work alongside/observe a clinical nurse specialist • Conduct departmental visits • Work alongside/observe other healthcare professionals	• Develop an understanding of specialist care • Gain exposure to a wider range of CLEs
Explore non-NHS services available in the local community	• Attend a day centre • Access support groups/charitable organisations	• Understand the broader context of health and social care • Gain an appreciation of service provision • Gain exposure to a wider range of CLEs
Look for experiences that cover both hospital and community settings	• Arrange a paramedic experience • Work alongside/observe a clinical nurse specialist	• Gain an appreciation of service provision • Gain exposure to a wider range of CLEs
Work with other health and social care professions	• Conduct departmental visits • Work alongside/observe other professionals	• Develop an understanding of the multidisciplinary team and how it functions • Gain exposure to a wider range of CLEs

on the practice setting and whether this is conducive to your learning. Useful questions to ask are:

➤ What is the organisation's view on the importance of nursing education?

➤ How well do organisational policies determine the scope of nursing education?

➤ What is the organisation's practice of supporting nursing education?

Frank's story (Mental Health nursing student)

'Definitely of the placements I have had so far the ones where the staffing was good numbers and staff were supported in their own development meant that I was welcomed and I really appreciated the time and effort the staff made to support my learning. It was great to hear what courses registered nurses were going on. Some even helped me with references or explaining stuff for an essay. Even just having a mentor who understood the pressure of being a student went a long way.'

Beth's story (Children's nursing student)

'It was pretty obvious for me when a placement did not really value students or learning. I did my best to be engaged and enthusiastic but when the culture was negative towards students and you are considered a hindrance it is not easy. I had to evaluate the placement and my comments were followed up. I am not sure if anything changed as a result but I appreciated my feedback was taken seriously.'

Richard's story (Adult nursing student)

'Me [sic] and my friends joke about on some placements we learn how not to be a mentor. I can see that the work demands on the nurses are hard but it is part of being a nurse to teach others and having such a negative attitude towards students is unfair. We don't just turn up wherever we like, the placements are given to us and we assume they are prepared and ready for us. When that is not the case it really impacts on my learning.'

Jojo's story (Learning Disabilities nursing student)

'The staff are really important as to how well my placement goes. Some of the best mentors are those that are really knowledgeable and at ease in their environment. The other important thing is when my mentor is supported by other staff covering for them to release them to teach and assess me. I can see they take my education seriously and the long term effect of this in making me a better nurse and someone who will want to act in the same way once I am registered.'

The type of placement, the teaching and learning opportunities and the organisational culture are all key attributes that will determine the effectiveness of the CLE. The final section of this chapter will look at the outcomes of the CLE.

The outcomes of the CLE

By being in the CLE you should experience several positive outcomes, namely the ongoing achievement of your learning outcomes, the further development of your practice and a continuing sense of fulfilment in your role as a student nurse.

Achievement of your learning outcomes

Each module that you study on the course has written learning outcomes. These guide the module content, the teaching and learning strategies and the assessment methods used in order that you achieve specific learning. These principles equally apply to your learning in practice. The key difference is that you will be expected to develop learning outcomes of your own in each placement. To support the formation and achievement of your learning outcomes you will be reliant on your mentor who has an insight not only into the profession but also into what learning can be gained within the CLE. Without working towards achieving explicit learning outcomes your learning during the placement will be ad hoc at best or meaningless at worst. Chapter 3 – 'How?' – provides specific guidance on how to devise learning outcomes with your mentor.

Understandably you will want to achieve all of your learning outcomes, however the CLE is a less dependable environment for learning compared to university. For example, you may find that planned learning opportunities or assessments have to be postponed. This can be a source of frustration or even anxiety for you as a student. Therefore, it is helpful to agree with your mentor in advance what to do in the event of unexpected changes or challenges to fulfilling your learning outcomes and document this in your **learning contract**. Ensure you review your learning contract regularly with your mentor to gauge the extent of your achievement of your learning outcomes. And remember you can always adapt any incomplete or unachieved learning outcomes into actions as part of an **action plan** to be followed up on your next placement(s).

It is important to not restrict the achievement of learning outcomes to any one individual CLE. As such in each new CLE, you should seek to maintain previously achieved learning outcomes. This reflects the inclusiveness of CLEs where reinforcement and repetition of your learning can really benefit your practice. Furthermore, the CLE will stretch you as you apply your prior learning to new clinical situations. Your mentor should be able to help you determine the transferability of your current learning. For example, you may already have learnt how to gain consent from a service user when administering their medication but in another CLE you may need to adapt this knowledge in the event of the person lacking capacity or as a result of your lack of familiarity with the medication.

The differences between each CLE will enable you to generate new learning outcomes. This continual refinement of your knowledge, skills and attitudes can be regarded as virtually limitless within CLEs. Most students view this as a powerful motivation for their ongoing learning and for registered nurses this often forms the basis of their **continuous professional development**. In Activity 2.5 you get to review you progress

---

Activity 2.5 Achievement of your learning outcomes – a review

Look at your self-assessments, learning contracts, reflections, feedback and completed assessments and answer the following questions:

- How would you describe your achievement to date?

- What are you basing this measure upon?

- What are you most proud of achieving?

- What do you still need to achieve?

- Are there any recurring themes for improvement?

- How have these themes been identified? Through personal reflection or feedback from a third party?

so far and identify the learning you have achieved and what you intend to achieve during the remainder of the course. It can often be a welcome surprise to also see the extent of your achievement.

By achieving your learning outcomes you will be developing your practice and hopefully feeling fulfilled in your role as a student nurse. These aspects are explored more fully in the following two sections.

Development of your practice

The learning you achieve in the CLE should not be considered in isolation from your learning at university. Neither should it be considered of more value or of greater relevance. It is the combination of these two areas alongside your independent study that underpins your learning. That said it is only within the CLE that you can fully demonstrate and evaluate the development of your practice.

The CLE acts as a means of triggering and testing your learning. Only through experiencing practice will you discover what it is like: how it makes you feel and what meaning you derive from the experience. By being in practice you will have the opportunity to combine your knowledge, skills and attitudes in real-time, real-life situations. You will be able to apply what you know and identify areas where you need to develop your learning further. For example, you may know it is important to gain informed consent, but are you aware of the process of how to do this and how it is documented? How is it different when you need consent in the case of a child or in an emergency?

Learning in practice is based on the idea of **experiential learning** developed by Kolb (2015). By experiencing practice you will interact with the environment, people and tasks. These experiences may or may not fit with your current knowledge level and ability. By reflecting on these experiences you can go on to construct greater knowledge and skills and a more meaningful understanding of yourself as a learner and your nursing practice. According to Kolb, in order for this learning to happen the learner should move through a four-stage cycle. Figure 2.2 presents the four-stage cycle and Activity 2.6 will help you understand how to work through each stage of the cycle.

Working through the stages of the cycle in order to learn from an experience may seem to you like an overly complex or unnecessary exercise. Or perhaps the idea of experiential learning is too abstract. However, as someone who is learning how to learn in practice it can be really helpful to adopt a more structured approach to your learning, as it will make your learning more obvious to you. You will be able to see how well you have understood something or the extent to which you have learnt it. It

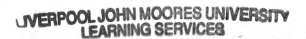

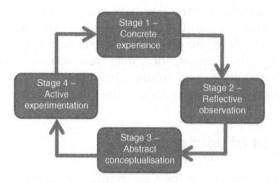

Figure 2.2   Kolb's (1984) experiential learning cycle

Kolb, David A., Experiential Learning: Experience As The Source Of Learning And Development, 2nd ed., ©2015. Reprinted by permission of Pearson Education, Inc., New York, New York.

Activity 2.6 Experiential Learning Cycle – working through each stage

Starting at Stage 1 – **concrete experience** refers to the actual experience you encounter or you have encountered in the past.

- List some of the concrete experiences you have had.
- Choose one and describe the experience.
- What actually happened?
- In this experience were you a participant or an observer?

Moving on to Stage 2 – **reflective observation** means you think about the experience.

- What were you doing, thinking, feeling in the experience?
- How do your past experiences compare to this current experience?
- What is similar or different between now and then?

Now you are ready for Stage 3 – **abstract conceptualisation** simply means you try to understand what you experienced.

- Why did this experience happen?
- Having reviewed the experience do you need to modify your existing knowledge, skills or attitudes?
- What do you need to add to or develop your current level of knowledge, skills or attitudes?

▶

◀

Finally you are at Stage 4 – **active experimentation** refers to testing out your understanding gained from the experience.

- Apply your learning to new experiences or reinterpreting past experiences
- What will I do when this experience happens again?
- What is the result of testing out your understanding?

This will lead to new experiences and repeating the cycle again.

will also prompt you to think about what you need to change or develop in your learning and get you to test out your new learning. The following stories are great examples of experiential learning. None refer to a formal process or adherence to a rigid structure but all reflect a cyclical approach that includes thinking about what happened, trying to understand what happened and testing out this understanding. Most importantly, all of the learning is derived from experiences in practice.

Alice's story (Children's nursing student)

'I was used to caring for children because of my past work experience but once I became a student nurse I knew I had to get more from what I was doing even if it was the same as before. We had had a lecture on pain management and when I was in practice I found it hard to assess a child's pain. I realised I needed to practice more and my mentor was really good at giving me lots of opportunities to do this. Each time I tried it out I thought how I could do it better. Sometimes I read more about it or asked my mentor or observed other people. It seemed like I was just concentrating on one small part of nursing but actually I was able to use the same skills in other ways such as learning how to write in the notes and review drug charts.'

Carmel's story (Mental Health nursing student)

'One of my mentors was really good at getting me to review what I had learnt in that shift. I would think back over the day and focus on what I did well first and then think a bit more about some of the things I struggled with. This became the plan for the next day to work out what was missing from my knowledge or skills and adding to it and then making sure I could try out my new learning as soon as possible.'

Wes's story (Adult nursing student)

'I really liked talking with my colleagues about placement. I would tell them about my day, what I did, how I got on. We would often end up talking about what we still had to learn and we'd share experiences and information on what helped us. I could then use this when I was back in practice.'

The primary goal of undertaking experiential learning is for you to develop safe and effective practice. This outcome is in part subject to how well you respond to variations to your practice, make adaptions to your practice and adjust to evolving practice.

Variations to your practice

When in the CLE, you may observe your mentor and/or other healthcare professionals demonstrating practice that differs from how you were taught. By all means ask questions and challenge, in a constructive way, any variations to practice that you observe. A good question to use in this situation is: 'I see that you are using a different technique to how I was taught; can you talk through it so I understand the differences?' As long as practice complies with policy and follows the evidence base, it is entirely reasonable to suppose that there may be different approaches that still achieve the same result of safe and effective practice. Clinicians may have developed strategies to make procedures more efficient or to accommodate service user preferences and to promote individualised care.

Issues will arise for you if either the standard of **best practice** presented at the university is exposed as erroneous or not up to date, or the credibility of your mentor or other clinicians is undermined by observing that they do not follow or may even be unaware of best practice. Ultimately, it will be up to you to determine what best practice *is* and to use your time in the CLE to assimilate this into your own practice. This will involve you undertaking research and critique of the evidence and information for a procedure or practice. Understanding the principles of a procedure or practice and knowing how to apply these when you encounter situations that differ from the norm or may be unfamiliar to you. And finally you will need to learn how to integrate this learning into your own practice to remain safe and effective.

Adapting your practice

You will need to learn to adapt your practice while continuing to ensure that service users receive the best quality care possible. The adaptions may be in response to:

> ➤ different CLEs, for example adapting your practice when on a community placement

> ➤ different service users, for example adapting your practice when a service user is not **concordant** or **compliant** with their treatment

> ➤ different staff, for example adapting your practice when working with staff other than your mentor

> ➤ different equipment, for example adapting your practice when you are using unfamiliar equipment

> ➤ different services, for example adapting your practice when there are service reconfigurations.

It can be difficult to cope with continually adapting or changing your practice. It is therefore helpful that during your course you develop **resilience** strategies; Chapter 3 – 'How?' – provides information on this. You will certainly need to get accustomed to working with change. As the NHS and its services have to be reflexive to meet demand you will find that specialisms may change overnight, and the placement you had been allocated is now an entirely different clinical area. At certain times of the year (most commonly referred to as winter pressures) the increase in service user admissions will mean hospitals may have to open up escalation wards. Likewise, services may be downsized/upgraded or NHS trusts may merge. In other CLEs, such as the community, the pressures are different but still very much an important consideration. For example, community colleagues find themselves having to frequently reprioritise their caseload in response to the addition of new service users and the clinical needs of all people on their caseload.

The standard to apply, when you have to adapt your practice, is to continue to provide best practice every time, for every service user. By way of an example, it is likely that you will have learnt early in your nursing education the importance of hand hygiene. However, once in practice how easy has it been for you to maintain effective hand hygiene? While there is no excuse for poor practice, part of what you will need to learn in the CLE is how to overcome difficulties in and compromises to achieving best practice.

Evolving your practice

The final key aspect in the development of your own practice is to recognise that nursing practice is evolving. As a student nurse the CLE should be a highly stimulating environment as you observe and potentially participate in studies, research trials and innovative practice. Similarly, you should observe how experience informs practice and prompts opportunities for ongoing learning. As a student you are considered a novice but the aim is for you to develop your practice so that you become a confident expert.

Fulfilment in your nursing role

While attending university, you will undoubtedly have had many inspiring lectures taught by vastly experienced lecturers who can expertly turn a complicated process or concept into something that is easy for you to understand. At the same time, you may also have sat through some less than engaging sessions and have been counting down the days until the next placement is due to start!

Either way, as a profession, nursing is practice-based and the best way to learn and understand in full the role of the nurse is to experience it first-hand. When in practice you will be working alongside professionals who will be able to teach you all they know, provide you with their guidance and share their 'tips of the trade'. And through this learning in the CLE it is hoped that you will gain a sense of fulfilment in your own emerging role as a nurse.

Frances' story (Children's nursing student)

'Initially I was learning tasks and I was enjoying this but I didn't feel much like a nurse. I realised I needed to focus everything I did though a nursing lens. Lots of things I learnt how to do I saw other staff doing including doctors, healthcare assistants. I started asking myself – what was my role as a nurse in the care of this child?'

Developing your own professional identity as a nurse is a significant outcome of the time you spend in the CLE. The experience of working alongside nurses and exercising an increasing level of autonomy in your practice will build your confidence and challenge any assumptions that you may have had about your own profession. Activity 2.7 will help you to consider the role of the nurse and how it is similar to or different from the roles of other healthcare professionals.

Activity 2.7 Whose role is it anyway?

When you are on placement consider the following:

- What are the roles that are shared by nurses and other healthcare professionals?
- What are the roles that are distinctive to nurses?
- Is this division in roles the same in every placement?
- What satisfies you, and why, about your nursing role?
- What frustrates you, and why, about your nursing role?

The intended outcomes of the CLE will enable you to develop both personally and professionally. The learning outcomes that you achieve in the CLE are personal to you, devised according to the stage you are at on the course, the placement type and your own learning needs. Yet by achieving and maintaining these learning outcomes you will also develop your professional knowledge, skills and attitudes. Through the experiential learning gained in the CLE you will be able to manage variations to your practice, as well as learn how to adapt and evolve your practice to uphold best practice for every service user, every time. Attaining this level of practice will provide you with a sense of fulfilment in your role both now as a student and in the future as a registered nurse.

Summary

This chapter has explored where you learn, providing you with a definition of the CLE as the place to apply your knowledge, skills and attitudes to prepare you for professional practice as a registered nurse. The model CLE is one in which, first, the prerequisites are met, ensuring that each placement is safe and supportive for nursing students and it has attained a level of quality assurance that safeguards the placement as a learning environment.

Secondly, the attributes of the CLE should ensure that each student experiences a diverse range of placement types within hospital and community settings, the student is exposed to sufficient teaching and learning opportunities, and the culture of the organisation has a commitment to foster and promote nursing education. Finally, as a result of attending the CLE the student should experience a number of positive outcomes including achievement of their learning outcomes, development of safe and effective practice and satisfaction in their emerging role as a nurse.

Yet you may not always experience a model CLE and borderline placements may mean your learning is restricted. This may be related to poor or unsafe practice, limitations in your mentor's ability or compromises to your supernumerary status. You will therefore need to use your time in the CLE to learn how to overcome your difficulties. This will include working alongside your mentor, reporting concerns, using the Assessment of Practice document as a guide for your learning, making full use of the learning opportunities available to you, including spoke experiences, and using the experiential learning approach.

Hopefully, despite these issues, your time in the CLE will enable you to develop your practice and your understanding of the profession. It will provide you with the facility of applying the knowledge that you gain at university to your practice in real-time, real-life situations. Through these experiences you will start to make connections in your understanding of seemingly disparate knowledge and to develop your clinical expertise to become a nurse.

Knowledge review

See Appendix 2 to compare your answers.

1. What are the prerequisites for a CLE?

2. Which placement types are present in all healthcare sectors – NHS, private and independent?

3. How would you define experiential learning?

4. How often should you provide best practice as a student nurse and once registered?

Further reading and resources

The following resources provide more detail about the Department of Health and the National Health Service:

Department of Health:

Health and Social Care Act (2012) – a UK law which establishes the structure and function of the NHS: http://www.legislation.gov.uk/ukpga/2012/7/contents/enacted

Department of Health policies on a wide range of health conditions and social care, for example children's health, dementia and health and social care integration: https://www.gov.uk/government/policies?keywords=&organisations%5B%5D=department-of-health

Essence of Care (2010) benchmark standards for best practice in a range of
    fundamental aspects of care, for example nutrition, patient safety, record
    keeping and so on: https://www.gov.uk/government/uploads/system/
    uploads/attachment_data/file/216691/dh_119978.pdf
Five Year Forward View (2014) – a report on the changing needs of healthcare
    and how to meet these demands in the future: https://www.england.nhs.uk/
    wp-content/uploads/2014/10/5yfv-web.pdf
The Five Year Forward View for Mental Health (2016) – a report from
    the independent Mental Health Taskforce on the provision of mental
    health services in England: https://www.england.nhs.uk/wp-content/
    uploads/2016/02/Mental-Health-Taskforce-FYFV-final.pdf
Raising the Bar. Shape of Caring: A Review of the Future Education and Training
    of Registered Nurses and Care Assistants (2015): https://www.hee.nhs.uk/
    sites/default/files/documents/2348-Shape-of-caring-review-FINAL.pdf
Leading Change, Adding Value (2016) a framework for nursing, midwifery
    and care staff for their role in leading and developing safe and effective
    care: https://www.england.nhs.uk/wp-content/uploads/2016/05/
    nursing-framework.pdf
Commissioning for Quality and Innovation – annually monitored targets for
    health and social care: https://www.england.nhs.uk/nhs-standard-contract/
    cquin/cquin-16-17/
National Institute for Health and Care Excellence (NICE) Quality Standards and
    Indicators – set out the priority areas for quality improvement in health and
    social care: https://www.nice.org.uk/standards-and-indicators

National Health Service (NHS):

Guide to the NHS on its structure and function: https://www.england.nhs.uk/
    wp-content/uploads/2014/06/simple-nhs-guide.pdf
NHS Constitution (2015) – a charter on the values of the NHS: https://www.
    gov.uk/government/uploads/system/uploads/attachment_data/file/480482/
    NHS_Constitution_WEB.pdf
NHS Outcomes Framework: https://www.gov.uk/government/publications/
    nhs-outcomes-framework-2016-to-2017
NHS Business Plan 2016–17: https://www.england.nhs.uk/wp-content/
    uploads/2016/03/bus-plan-16.pdf

3
How?

Learning outcomes

After reading and completing the activities in this chapter you will be able to:

➢ Identify the principles of how you learn.

➢ Develop solutions to the challenges you will encounter in your practice learning.

➢ Reflect on your preferred learning style(s).

➢ Recognise the range of learning strategies available to support your learning in practice.

Generally, within the first few shifts of working with your mentor they will ask you something along the lines of what you want to get out of the placement or what you would like to learn. But have you ever been asked by your mentor *how* you learn? And what would you say if you were? If you struggle to answer the former question it may be because you have not spent enough time working out the answer to the latter. Try out Activity 3.1 to get you thinking about how you learn.

Activity 3.1 What are your assumptions about how you learn?

Think about a time when you had to learn something new, for example driving a car, using new technology, learning a language?

• What did you expect the learning experience to be like?

• Why was it important to learn this?

• How did you go about learning this?

• How successful was your learning?

How you learn will often govern what you learn. For example, if you learn best by observing but you have had no opportunity to do this before being asked to complete a task, the level of your learning is likely to be limited – even if you know the importance of learning how to do this task. The extent of your learning can be compounded further by the added dimension of where the learning takes place. Learning in practice is a very different and often unfamiliar learning environment compared to university.

Table 3.1 lists the similarities and differences between learning at university and learning in practice. You will be familiar with how you learn at university because it will most likely parallel your previous learning experiences. For example, when you attend a lecture you know: where to go, what time it starts and when it is expected to finish, and what the lecture will be about; you may even have had the lecture notes in advance, and you will have chosen to take notes or just sit and listen according to your preferred learning style.

Transport yourself into the **clinical learning environment** (CLE) and invariably how you learn in practice will be completely different to your learning at university, bringing with it unique challenges and obstacles. Key differences include the absence of a timetable with the teaching planned out; no one able/willing to teach you; and the learning opportunities such as they are often being ad hoc and unstructured. Even the physical space is less conducive to learning – for example, it is unlikely that you will have a desk to lean on to take notes – you may have limited or no access to the internet and nowhere to plug in your laptop. Beyond these variations, a fundamental difference, between practice and university is that the focus in practice is not on you and your learning but

Table 3.1 Similarities and differences between learning at university and learning in practice

How you learn at university	How you learn in practice
Attend lectures, seminars, workshops	Attend practice
Complete independent study	Complete independent study
Majority of learning is planned by the teacher	Majority of learning is planned by the student
Ratio of student to lecturer is >1:1	Ratio of student to mentor is 1:1
Refer to experiences	Undertake experiences
Reflect on experiences	Reflect on experiences
Exam, essay, presentation assessments	Competency and skill assessments
Familiar, controlled environment	Unfamiliar, dynamic environment

rather on the service user and their care. This is somewhat of a paradox as the primary reason for you to be in practice is to learn how to care for the service user but the very act of caring for them can limit and challenge your learning.

Rob's story (Mental Health nursing student)

'I guess the biggest frustration and the thing that causes me and my fellow students the most anxiety is having to chase our mentors to get the assessments completed. Mentors have good intentions but time just disappears. The mentor gets called away to help with something or the day is just so busy and our plans get sidetracked.'

Katie's story (Children's nursing student)

'It was a big adjustment for me figuring out how to make the most of my placements. I had been told to prepare and ask questions but when you are faced with all these new experiences and everyone else doing their work and being so good at it you can feel overwhelmed and wonder, how will I learn everything? I realised I needed to treat my placements differently to being at uni; I couldn't have the same way of learning. I started doing simple things like using my phone to take pictures of how to set up a trolley or making the most of the 1:1 time with mentors.'

Charlie's story (Learning Disabilities nursing student)

'Being in practice is great and you learn lots but sometimes it does feel a bit too random. I chat with my colleagues and they are learning different things. This may be because of the type of placement or the mentor but I do wonder if I will get to learn that.'

Being in practice can be interesting and exciting but it can also be a difficult and anxiety-provoking experience. Set this against the activity and demands of each placement and somehow you are expected to learn how to become a nurse. By establishing the principles of how you learn in order to maximise and overcome the challenges to your learning in practice, you will develop your own strategies and ways of learning. The first chapter provided the rationale as to *why* you learn in practice and the second chapter explored *where* your practice learning takes place. In this third chapter you will recognise *how* you learn in order to achieve *what* you need to learn in Chapter 4. The nature of how you learn is based on the following three principles: first, you have the ability to learn; secondly you can learn in different ways; and thirdly you are responsible for your own learning.

You have the ability to learn

Think back to what you have already achieved in order to become a student nurse studying at university for a degree and professional registration. You were accepted on the course because you demonstrated an ability to learn and the potential over the next three years to further develop your learning. Learning, therefore, is the ability to relate new information to previously acquired knowledge. The first of the three principles of learning is based on the premise that, given your readiness to learn, expressing the attributes of a learner and receiving the necessary support for your learning, you have the ability to learn.

Readiness to learn

Your readiness to learn is linked to the concept of motivation. Motivation acts as the stimulus for you to learn, yet it is unlikely that your level of motivation will remain constant throughout the course. You will experience many different circumstances and events that will alter your motivation to learn. This may include changes in your personal life, success or failure in your studies and how you are affected by your practice experiences. As a student encountering a different clinical setting with each new placement it can be difficult to maintain your motivation as you may feel that you are back at square one again, that is, you have to learn new routines, new terminology and meet new people each and every time. Activity 3.2 will help you gauge your current level of motivation for learning; it may be helpful to compare the outcome of this activity if you were to repeat it at various times throughout your course.

The last two questions, in Activity 3.2 – 'What motivates/demotivates you about this experience?' – are intended to elicit the external and internal drivers of your motivation. External drivers are factors outside of you, whereas internal drivers are those inherent within you that will influence the degree of motivation you have to learn.

Activity 3.2 How motivated are you?

What are your three most significant clinical experiences to date?

For each experience complete the table:

What can you now do?	What can you still not do?
_____	_____
_____	_____
What do you now know?	**What do you still not know?**
_____	_____
_____	_____
What motivates you about this experience?	**What demotivates you about this experience?**
_____	_____
_____	_____
_____	_____

Examples of external drivers:

➤ encountering experiences that challenge your knowledge, skills and attitudes

➤ having clear expectations/instructions of what and how you are to learn

➤ receiving feedback on how effective your learning is

➤ upholding patient safety and well-being

➤ maintaining effective teamwork and interprofessional communication.

Examples of internal drivers:

➤ your curiosity to learn and understand

➤ the perceived benefit to you of learning

➢ your understanding of the importance of being able to know/do something correctly

➢ the satisfaction/sense of achievement you derive from learning.

Look again at Activity 3.2 to identify whether your answers for the last two questions reflect internal and/or external drivers. Your motivation to learn in practice will invariably be a combination of both factors. For example, you may have the satisfaction of being able to answer fully a service user's question (internal) and your mentor may give you some feedback to help you work on an area of nursing practice that you need to improve (external). The risk is that what you have to learn, in order to become a nurse, may hold no motivation for you either internally or externally. Therefore, you may become demotivated if you see no value or purpose in your learning. In Activity 3.3 you will identify the Nursing and Midwifery Council (NMC) competencies and then answer some questions designed to foster your motivation to learn how to achieve these in your nursing education.

Activity 3.3 NMC Competencies?

Look through the NMC competencies and skills; these are available in the Standards for Pre-registration Nursing Education (NMC 2010) but may also be stated in your **Assessment of Practice document.**

- For each competency/skill identify, what are the benefits to you and others of achieving this competency?

- For each competency/skill identify, why it is important to you and others to achieve this competency?

- Do you have a sense of achievement when you successfully complete each competency/skill? If yes, why? If no, why not?

The attributes of a learner

Your learning is not just dependent on the level of your motivation. Overarching this is displaying the right attributes of a learner to ensure that you derive meaning from your experiences in practice. As a student you should be developing the following attributes:

➢ **Integration** – this means seeking out opportunities to apply your *current* knowledge, skills and attitudes into your practice. This will reinforce your learning and help you to identify your learning needs.

➢ **Transition** – this means transferring your *current* knowledge, skills and attitudes from one placement to the next and from each academic year to the next. This will avoid the risks of learning in isolation and devaluing your learning.

➢ **Assimilation** – this means adapting and using your *new* knowledge, skills and attitudes in your practice. This will ensure you continue to develop your learning.

➢ **Progression** – this means your learning should advance your practice. Your learning should move you on from foundational skills in order to become an autonomous practitioner.

Table 3.2 presents the intrinsic qualities that underpin the attributes you require to make your learning successful. The table also includes a column with a cross-reference to where you can find further information on these qualities in this chapter.

Emotional intelligence

Alongside having an IQ, a key factor in your learning is your emotional intelligence (EQ). This means the extent to which you have an

Table 3.2   The intrinsic qualities of a learner

Intrinsic qualities – what you have	Further information
Motivation/focus	See section on 'Readiness to learn'
Questioning skills	See section on 'Strategies for learning' – Reinforcement of an experience
Ability to manage your anxiety	See section on 'Mechanisms to support you' – Managing your anxiety
Communication skills	See section on 'The attributes of a learner' – Emotional intelligence
Confidence/assertiveness	See section on 'The attributes of a learner' – Emotional intelligence
Critical thinking skills	See section on 'Strategies for learning' – Reinforcement of an experience
Reflective skills	See section on 'Strategies for learning' – Reflection on an experience
Flexibility/adaptability to change	See section on 'The attributes of a learner' – Emotional intelligence
Resilience skills	See section on 'Mechanisms to support you' – Building your resilience

Rose's story (Learning Disabilities nursing student)

'I thought I would find each new placement challenging, but as I built up my experience and understood more about my role I was able to prepare better for the next placement. I still had difficulties but I realised I could overcome these. Sometimes this was because I sorted it out or because I asked. Definitely, asking for help should not be seen as a weakness.'

understanding of yourself and how you interact with others. Being more aware of your EQ will improve your confidence levels and your communication skills which will enhance your learning in practice. The two elements of EQ are personal and social competence.

Personal competence is made up of:

➢ *Self-awareness* – of your thoughts and feelings. When you are in practice acknowledge your thoughts and feelings and how these might impact on your behaviour.

➢ *Self-confidence* – in who you are and your abilities. When you are in practice rather than thinking 'W*ill I be able to do this?'* affirm that you are a student and your abilities will grow with experience and support.

➢ *Self-management* – taking responsibility and being adaptable to change. When you are in practice recognise that you can change your behaviour to reduce stress and improve your performance.

Social competence comprises:

➢ Empathy – awareness and understanding of other's feelings and concerns. When in practice ensure you are non-judgemental and avoid assumptions. Respect people as individuals and be willing to listen to their story.

➢ Social skills – seeking to communicate clearly. When in practice be assertive (not aggressive), own your communication, use 'I' rather than 'you' to explain the effect of other people's actions on you.

Challenges to your learning

Clinical practice will present a variety of challenges for you that can impact on your learning. These may include your inexperience, a disconnection between your time at university and in practice, and the difficulties in applying nursing theory to practice. These issues can be compounded further when you receive little or no supervision or support from your mentor. Even the nature of the CLE being dynamic, changeable and unpredictable can lead to difficulties in making sense of your experiences in practice. Furthermore, the variability in placements will affect whether you will be able to achieve your learning needs. You will also be subject to managing your expectations and assumptions, about what it means to be a nurse, against the realities and demands of clinical practice.

Students have reported the following issues with their learning in practice:

➤ not being recognised as part of the profession

➤ the transient nature of being a student

➤ not feeling welcome or not accepted

➤ mentors not divulging/withholding their knowledge or expertise

➤ the tension between what is taught and what is practised

➤ having to focus on completing the Assessment of Practice document

➤ issues around status and feeling powerless

➤ organisational constraints (such as staffing and resourcing) which challenge supernumerary status

➤ conflict in priorities between learning and the demands of clinical practice

➤ managing different shift patterns/clinical settings/teams

➤ lacking a sense of belonging.

(Henderson and Cooke 2012)

Here are some questions to ask yourself when you encounter difficulties in practice:

➤ What is the nature of the difficulty?

➤ How might this difficulty impact on my learning?

➤ If you have had any positive experiences what worked and why? How can you apply this to your current situation?

➤ What is your role and responsibility in managing this difficulty?

➤ What is the role and responsibility of your mentor in managing this difficulty?

➤ What do you need to manage/sustain you in your learning in practice?

➤ Who do you need to help you manage/sustain you in your learning?

➤ What intrinsic qualities do you have that enable your learning?

➤ What extrinsic qualities does your mentor have that enable your learning?

Becoming a nurse will mean you should respond professionally in all situations even if they cause you stress or distress. It would be concerning if a nurse was unable to work out a strategy to cope or the strategies they employed led to unprofessional or unsafe practice.

Receiving support

Despite being highly motivated, having the right attributes, developing the intrinsic qualities of a learner and being emotionally intelligent you will still need support to manage the challenges to your learning. By accessing the available support your learning will greatly benefit. At the start of the course it is usual to require more support but as you progress this level of support will most likely reduce over time. However, you should have a low threshold for seeking support regardless of which year you are in or the extent of support your peers are receiving. A change in your circumstances may warrant receiving a level of support higher than you had anticipated.

Studying on a nursing course is demanding as it requires a significant commitment, in terms of your time. As a result, this often leaves less time and energy for maintaining work–life balance. Coupled with the demands of the course many students unfortunately experience events in their personal lives which have an adverse impact on their ability to continue studying. Without effective support your learning in practice will be impaired, directly impacting on how well you can attain the required knowledge, skills and attitudes. See Box 3.1 for the 10 most common

---

Box 3.1 The 10 most common reasons students access support in practice

1. **The student has difficulties with their mentor** – this can be due to mentor absence/sickness, the mentor leaving and not being replaced, the mentor's workload/commitments or a personality clash between the mentor and the student.

▶

◄

2. **The student has unexpected absence/sickness** – students become concerned about the impact the absence will have on their recorded hours and their ability to complete the practice-based assessments.

3. **The student has difficult accessing/organising learning** – this can be due to the type of placement or mentor/student-related issues such as absence/sickness, workload/commitments, motivation, professional behaviour, time management, lack of preparation, lack of understanding of the Assessment of Practice documentation.

4. **The student has difficulties with completing their assessments** – this can be due to the type of placement or mentor/student-related issues such as absence/ sickness, workload/commitments, motivation, professional behaviour, time management, lack of preparation, lack of understanding of assessment processes and the Assessment of Practice documentation.

5. **The student has personal issues affecting their practice** – students may have personal issues related to themselves, family or friends which may impact on their attendance, motivation, professional behaviour.

6. **The student has concerns about practice** – students should raise concerns about an aspect of care or a significant incident they observed.

7. **The student has failed an assessment** – students may be distressed due to failing and concerned about the impact this will have on their course progression.

8. **The student has sustained an injury/been involved in an incident** – students may have suffered an injury, for example needle-stick, or became involved in an incident which requires reporting and follow-up care.

9. **The student has academic work to complete while on placement** – students may have additional pressure to complete outstanding academic work while on placement.

10. **The student has anxiety related to practice** – students may have been involved in an adverse/distressing event for which they require debriefing and possible removal from the specific placement.

reasons students access support while on placement. How many do you identify with?

People to support you

The relationships you have with your mentors and your peers will probably be the most significant form of support you will receive and, in Chapter 5 – 'Who?', the different roles of people you will encounter in practice is explored in more detail. In this section the supportive roles undertaken by staff at university and in practice will be presented.

> **Gavin's story (Adult nursing student)**
>
> 'I had to be okay with asking for help; being an adult I was used to doing everything for myself and I was a bit reluctant to admit I couldn't do it all. Sometimes I had to ask a few people before I got the help but once I was supported it was much better and I wished I had asked sooner.'

Being an adult learner you can wrongly assume that you should manage every issue or difficulty on your own. While the people at university and in practice may not be able to take away the circumstances that you as a student are experiencing they can help to alleviate the pressures of the course and assist you in better managing your practice learning. Table 3.3 provides a list of staff and their responsibilities in supporting you.

Table 3.3 University and practice support roles and responsibilities

Role	Location	Responsibilities
Course Lead	University	• Quality assures placements
		• Agrees any change to your practice hours – e.g. if you have an un/expected absence
Placement Team	University	• Allocates placements for students
		• Records student attendance
Personal Tutor	University	• Supports your personal well-being, academic studies and professional development
Module Lead[1]	University	• Provides clinical skills sessions, simulations and resources to support practice learning
		• Advises students on completion of the assessment of practice book
		• Coordinates mandatory training – e.g. moving and handling and basic life support
Link Lecturer[2]	University	• Advises students and mentors on practice-related issues
		• Conducts educational audits
		• Troubleshoots student absences/issues
Disability Liaison Lecturer	University	• Develops learning support plans for students while in practice
		• Facilitates implementation of reasonable adjustments in practice
Student Services	University	• Advice and counselling service for students

Table 3.3 *Continued*

Role	Location	Responsibilities
Mentor	Practice	• Facilitates student learning and assessment in practice
Practice Educator[3]	Practice	• Provides educational resources and training to staff and students
Practice Education Facilitator[4]	Practice	• Coordinates placement provision • Conducts educational audits • Provides mentor updates • Troubleshoots mentor absences/issues
Occupational Health	Practice	• Confirm clearance for fitness to practice • Advise on health-related issues in practice

1. Module Lead is an academic staff member who leads the module linked to your assessment of practice.
2. Link Lecturer is an academic staff member who has a facilitative role in supporting students and mentors in practice. Alternative titles include Link Tutor, Practice Liaison Lecturer and Practice Tutor.
3. Practice Educator is a clinical staff member who is responsible for the education of staff within their clinical speciality, for example Critical Care, Forensic Unit, Theatres and so on.
4. Practice Education Facilitator is a clinical staff member who coordinates student placements in conjunction with the placement team. Alternative titles include Placement Coordinator and Student Education Lead.

As Table 3.3 shows there are several different staff who you can contact for support covering a host of reasons. While there are many avenues of support open to you while you are in the CLE your most immediate support will always be your mentor. It is their role to guide and support you in practice. But if your need for support concerns the mentor it may not be appropriate to discuss it with them. You may then decide to approach other practice-based staff. If your placement is in a specialist department check to see if a dedicated practice educator is in post who can act as a point of contact. It is also worth remembering that each department will have a nursing manager or lead who has overall responsibility for the practice in that area, and who can be considered as another worthwhile contact. Many clinical settings will have a central team of practice education facilitators (PEFs) who oversee the provision of clinical education, and whose contact details you should make sure you know.

As well as, or instead of, practice-based staff are those staff available within the HEI setting. As a student you will have access to module leads, professional practice leads, the course lead and personal tutors. The NMC (2010) also advocates the role of a link lecturer, or equivalent title. Such individuals are university-based staff who have a responsibility to liaise regularly with the practice setting, to manage practice-based queries and issues and to complete educational audits in partnership with practice.

Earlier in the chapter, Table 3.4 lists the extrinsic requirements that you need from practice and university staff to facilitate your learning.

Table 3.4   Extrinsic requirements

Extrinsic – what you need
Welcoming and valuing you as a person
Acknowledging you as a learner
Integrating you into the team
Establishing clear expectations of you
Facilitating your learning opportunities
Facilitating interprofessional learning
Articulating to you how they make clinical decisions
Being an effective role model for you
Giving you feedback on your progress
Providing guidance to you on how to transfer your learning

Mechanisms to support you

By recognising in advance what might compromise your practice learning you can learn how to handle these difficulties even before you encounter them and become more confident in the event of experiencing issues in practice. It is important that you acknowledge the reality of your concerns but also that you adopt an attitude of wanting to resolve these concerns rather than ignoring or dismissing them. This does not necessarily mean working out your solutions in isolation; as the previous section shows there are many other people with specific roles as well as your colleagues and peers who are able to support you. Be aware that this assistance may include challenging your current knowledge/experience/ability or helping you to avoid making assumptions.

You will also need to develop a range of support strategies that safeguard you against feeling overwhelmed or unable to cope so that you can continue to learn in practice. Building your resilience to stressors, managing your anxiety and devising a learning support plan can be considered as the key support mechanisms available to you in practice.

Building your resilience

Resilience is about overcoming difficult situations and more recently it is also understood to mean working towards changing the difficult situation as well (Hart and Heaver 2013). The time you spend in practice will require and reinforce your resilience. For example, you may experience days on placement where you feel you only just managed to get through them and the last thing you then want to do is go in the next day. But by going in the next day this can be an important step in overcoming your difficulties and building up your resilience.

Figure 3.1 is a resilience framework which highlights the key principles for supporting and maintaining your resilience.

You will note from the framework that your ability to be resilient, to bounce back, combines personal and social activities. By reinforcing positive character traits, adopting self-help exercises, accepting constructive feedback and engaging in social events you build up your resilience. While you are in practice you can test out these various approaches and use them to support and strengthen your learning. Details on resilience are available in the 'Further reading and resources' section at the end of this chapter.

Christopher's story (Children's nursing student)

'I really struggled to cope with the shift work when I first started and I had to figure out a way of managing as I was starting to be late for shifts and not making a good impression. I chatted with my friends and realised they were a bit more organised and also negotiated an easier working pattern with their mentors. By having the confidence to speak with my mentor, who responded really well, I had a better run of shifts which meant I was more focused and things started to click. I looked forward to going on placement and being there to learn.'

Managing your anxiety

Stress is a part of everyday life but sometimes your experience of stress can lead to feelings of anxiety. By recognising the causes of stress in your life, especially on placement, you will be better able to work towards reducing your anxiety. If you are finding you have significant physical and emotional responses to stress then it is best to contact your GP and discuss these issues further with a professional.

Practice is often the part of the course that students like most but it can also be stressful. Some of the stressors that are reported by nursing students include their first clinical placement, undertaking procedures, completing practice assessments and establishing relationships with staff and service users (Nelwati and Plummer 2013). Other stressors result from experiencing feelings of powerlessness and uncertainty or lacking competence.

Interestingly, stress can have favourable as well as unfavourable consequences for nursing students, as it can act as a catalyst for more useful

Resilience Framework (Adults) – Copyright Hart, Blincow & Cameron (adapted from original) www.boingboing.org.uk					
	BASICS	**BELONGING**	**LEARNING**	**COPING**	**CORE SELF**
SPECIFIC APPROACHES	Good enough housing	Find somewhere to belong	Make work & learning as successful as possible	Understanding boundaries and keeping within them	Instil a sense of hope
		Help understand place in the world, & that others may face similar situations		Being brave	
	Enough money to live	Tap into good influences (e.g. peer support)	Engage mentors	Identifying & solving problems (reduce self blame and guilt)	Promote understanding of others
	Being safe	Keep relationships going (e.g. educator/ support partners/carers/family)			
		The more healthy relationships the better	Map out career or life plan	Putting on rose-tinted glasses (reframing/reappraising)	Help the person to know her/himself
	Access & transport	Take what you can from relationships where there is some hope		Fostering their interests	
	Healthy diet	Get together people the person can count on	Help self-organisation	Calming down & self-soothing (support reflection, not feeling overwhelmed by illness)	Help the person take responsibility for her/himself (self-advocacy)
		Responsibilities & obligations			
	Exercise and fresh air	Focus on good times and places	Highlight achievements	Remember tomorrow is another day	Foster talents
	Enough sleep	Make sense of where the person has come from		Lean on others when necessary	
	Leisure & work occupations	Predict a good experience of someone or something new	Develop life skills		There are tried and tested treatments for specific problems, use them
		Make friends and mix		Have a laugh	
NOBLE TRUTHS					
	ACCEPTING Interpersonal skills, empathy	**CONSERVING** Interpersonal skills, trust	**COMMITMENT** Ongoing support issues		**ENLISTING** Self (eg not passive), family, friends, mental health professionals, GP

Figure 3.1 Resilience framework

Reprinted by permission of Hart, A. http://www.boingboing.org.uk

and successful learning or it can impede learning. Therefore, controlling and adjusting the level of anxiety experienced is most important (Ranjbar 2016). Alongside undertaking **reflection** of your practice, there are numerous techniques available to train yourself to focus on calming thoughts which will alleviate your feelings of anxiety (see Appendix 7 for an example of a mindfulness exercise). If you are already feeling anxious, making small, simple adjustments can make a big difference:

➤ Assessments are not designed to stress you out! If you are unable to achieve at first attempt you will be given feedback and further opportunities to achieve. It is okay to not achieve first time; learning from mistakes is still learning.

➤ Have a change of scenery – go outside, go for a walk, meet a friend (make friends).

➤ Eat well, drink well and sleep well.

➤ Try a mini meditation – breathe in deeply, count to five and exhale slowly. Repeat five times.

➤ Engage in positive self-talk to help build self-confidence.

➤ Face your fears head on. Avoiding stressful situations can reinforce anxiety.

➤ Don't try to be perfect. Remind yourself that your best is something to be proud of.

➤ Watch, listen or read something that makes you laugh out loud to relieve tension and focus on positive thoughts and feelings.

Activity 3.4 will show you that you are not alone in having concerns, and help you learn from how others manage their stress.

Activity 3.4 What do others do to manage their stress and anxiety?

Ask your peers/mentors what makes them feel stressed? Is it the same or different for you?

Ask what your peers/mentors do about feeling stressed?

How can you adopt their methods as your own?

Aisha's story (Learning Disabilities nursing student)

'I've felt I've been out of my depth and thought nobody ever debriefs you on these things…But the reflective groups we have at uni have helped and also working through issues with my mentor. I wouldn't say I feel overly stressed but sometimes things stay with me and I need to process it more.'

Devising your learning support plan

Evidence shows that nursing courses have a higher ratio of students who will have specific learning needs (Howlin and Halligan 2014). National legislation, namely 'The Equality Act 2010', obliges HEIs to facilitate inclusive practices for all students and prohibits discrimination against individuals with a disability. You would be deemed to have a disability if you have a physical or mental impairment that has a substantial and/or long-term negative effect on your ability to complete normal daily activities. Students who disclose a disability or a protected characteristic (see Box 3.2 for examples) should be supported by the university disability services who will conduct an individual academic needs assessment.

Box 3.2 Examples of disclosed disabilities and protected characteristics

Disclosed disabilities:

- learning impairment – for example, dyslexia
- visual/hearing impairment
- physical disability – for example, dyspraxia
- mental ill health – for example, anxiety or depression

Protected characteristics:

- age
- disability
- gender reassignment
- marriage and civil partnership

▶

◀

- pregnancy and maternity

- race

- religion or belief

- sex

- sexual orientation

As 50% of pre-registration nursing education is completed in practice, the CLE poses unique challenges to students that may not be addressed by an academic learning support plan alone. A learning support plan for practice should also be written in conjunction with the student, student services and practice staff. It should detail the requirements needed to support the student's learning while on placement and be subject to regular review. These requirements are more correctly termed **reasonable adjustments** and need not be onerous or complicated. Often the implementation of reasonable adjustments in practice can be advantageous to all students, not just those for whom it has been designed to benefit.

The Royal College of Nursing has produced guidance for mentors and students on developing reasonable adjustments – see the 'Further reading and resources' section at the end of this chapter for the link. Table 3.5 presents a list of common adjustments to support student

Table 3.5 Common reasonable adjustments to support practice learning

Time	Reading and writing	Practice
• Allow additional time after handover for student to plan activities • Allow time for the student to complete patient notes and record information • Encourage student to keep a 'to-do list' • Help student to prioritise tasks in the time available	• Provide a list of commonly used terminology and abbreviations • Allow use of health-related apps and spelling/dictionary apps • Provide regular written and verbal feedback on student performance • Allow student to refer to notes/lists when assessing knowledge • Provide handover sheet in advance	• Avoid allocating 12-hour shifts • Plan shift pattern/allocation in advance to enable student to know who they are working with • Allow student time to plan activities • Offer opportunities to practise in stages • Break down complex skills into 'bite-sized' sections

.... (student name) is a 1st / 2nd /

3rd year student completing the BSc (Hons) Nursing Course. The student

has been cleared as fit for practice by the Occupational Health Department

and is to be supported in practice with the following reasonable

adjustments:

Completed by: ....(name and designation)

Signature: ....Date: ....

Student signature: ....

Date: ....

Review date: ....

Review comments:

Figure 3.2 Practice learning support plan (template)

learning and Figure 3.2 is a learning support plan template that can be
adapted for your use.

Having established that the first principle of how you learn is based on
your ability to learn, which incorporates having a good level of motivation, possessing the right attributes and seeking support in order to better
facilitate and overcome difficulties learning in practice, the next principle
will explore the ways you can learn in practice.

You learn in different ways

You will hold your own beliefs about what it means to be experienced and knowledgeable, and what it takes to become so – as individuals have different dispositions and approaches to their learning. This is more commonly termed your learning style. It is unlikely that during your time in practice you are conscious of which learning style you are implementing. However, the advantages to knowing your own learning style(s) are the following:

➤ you will be able to increase your awareness of how you learn which will lead to improvements in your learning

➤ you will be better able to make your learning style fit learning opportunities

➤ you will be able to strengthen weaker learning styles

➤ you will be better able to overcome difficulties encountered with your learning

➤ you will be better able to manage your mentor's style of teaching.

In this section three different groups of learning styles will be presented. Each grouping will include a definition and suggested learning strategies best suited to that style of learning. The groupings are not mutually exclusive; therefore, it is possible that, for example, a pragmatist (a learning style from group 1) may also be a visual learner (a learning style from group 2) and a philosopher (a learning style from group 3). While everyone has different styles of learning an important characteristic of effective learning is that it is modifiable. Even if you identify with one style in particular be prepared to work on adopting other learning styles as well.

Learning styles group 1 – activist, theorist, pragmatist and reflector

The four distinct learning styles in this group – activist, theorist, pragmatist and reflector – were identified by Peter Honey and Alan Mumford (Honey and Mumford 2006). Table 3.6 provides the common attributes and the most appropriate learning strategies for each particular learning style. To determine your own learning style complete the Honey and Mumford Learning Styles Questionnaire – see the 'Further reading and resources' section for a link to the questionnaire. Even if you have completed this questionnaire before it can be a helpful

Table 3.6 Honey and Mumford learning styles

Learning style	Attributes	Best suited learning strategies
Activist	• Activists learn by experience • Activist require an open mind • Activists prefer to involve themselves fully in experiences	• practice experience • problem solving • group discussion
Theorist	• Theorists learn by understanding the theory behind the experience • Theorists require information about the experience • Theorists prefer to analyse and synthesise experiences	• stories/quotes • background information/models • discussion
Pragmatist	• Pragmatists learn by testing out learning on new experiences • Pragmatists require concrete rather than abstract examples/experiences • Pragmatists prefer time to process learning experiences	• case studies • problem solving • discussion • skills rehearsal
Reflector	• Reflectors learn by observing and thinking about experiences • Reflectors require distance from the experience • Reflectors prefer to view the experience from different perspectives	• paired discussions • self-analysis questionnaires • observation • feedback/coaching

exercise to compare your previous result with your current learning style. Is it the same or different?

Your questionnaire result will also show you whether you are biased towards one style in particular or whether your score is applied evenly across all learning styles. The latter is a better outcome as no one style is superior to another and all learning styles are necessary for comprehensive learning. By mapping the Honey and Mumford learning styles onto the four stages of Kolb's experiential learning model (refer to Chapter 2 – 'Why?') you can see that each learning style applies to a specific stage of the learning cycle (see Figure 3.3). The concrete experience stage is aligned to the activist learning style, and to move from a concrete experience to the reflective observation stage you would be required to become a reflector. To optimise the abstract conceptualisation stage you would use the theorist learning style, and being a pragmatist suits the active experimentation stage. The most successful learners, therefore, are those that can adapt their learning style according to the stage of the learning cycle they are at.

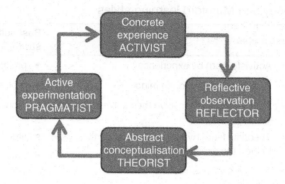

Figure 3.3   Diagram of Honey and Mumford learning styles mapped onto Kolb's experiential learning cycle

Learning styles group 2 – visual, aural, read/write and kinaesthetic

The Honey and Mumford learning styles describe characteristics of learning, whereas these four learning styles represent particular modes of learning, that is, people learn best by visual, aural, reading/written or practical methods. Of the total population approximately 22% will be visual learners, 26% aural learners, 24% read/write learners and 28% kinaesthetic learners (Fleming 2001). A brief summary of each mode is presented along with the most beneficial approaches to learning in this manner.

Visual learners have a preference for learning using information that is presented in visual format. When in practice visual learner's benefit from:

➢ observing practice – for example, clinical and non-clinical activities

➢ accessing visual material – for example, flow charts, documentation, algorithms

➢ e-learning activities – for example, mandatory training, specialist education.

Aural learners have a preference for learning using information that is spoken or heard. When in practice aural learners benefit from:

➢ questioning – for example, being able to ask/be asked questions

➢ discussion – for example, planning care with the multidisciplinary team and service user

➤ receiving verbal feedback – for example, from their mentor

➤ attending meetings or study days – for example, multidisciplinary meetings, morbidity and mortality meetings, in-house training, mandatory training, specialist education.

Read/write learners have a preference for learning using information that is produced in printed form. When in practice read/write learners benefit from:

1. Accessing written material to read – for example, documentation, summary of product characteristics, patient leaflets, policy, guidelines.

2. Writing and completing documentation – for example, care plan, observation charts.

3. E-learning activities – for example, mandatory training, specialist education.

4. Receiving written feedback – for example, from mentor.

Kinaesthetic learners have a preference for learning using information that is derived from tangible experiences. When in practice kinaesthetic learners benefit from:

➤ Participating in practice – for example, clinical and non-clinical activities.

➤ Departmental visits – for example, escorting a service user for investigations or treatment.

➤ Skills rehearsal – for example, problem solving and deciding how to complete a clinical activity.

Joanna's story (Adult nursing student)

'I liked being immersed in practice; it made my learning real and helped me to remember all the different things I needed to know. I also took lots of information home to read like the paper that came with the medications in the box and patient information leaflets. This made it easier to answer patients' questions as I had the right information to give them.'

Learning styles group 3 – analyser, organiser, philosopher and reflector

The final grouping of learning styles aims to optimise your learning by enabling you to tailor the learning style to the learning opportunity (Fleming 2011). To identify the best learning style to use you need to consider your position along two continuums:

➤ The processing continuum – that is, your approach to this learning opportunity: to get involved (*doing*) or just to stand back and observe (*watching*)?

➤ The perceiving continuum – that is, your response to this learning opportunity: to consider it (thinking) or to get a sense of it (feeling)?

For each given learning opportunity you will move along the two continuums. Therefore, your learning will be characterised by any of the following combinations:

➤ *Doing* and *thinking* – this would make you an analyser.

➤ *Doing* and *feeling* – this would make you an organiser.

➤ *Watching* and *thinking* – this would make you a philosopher.

➤ *Watching* and *feeling* – this would make you a reflector.

Figure 3.4 plots the learning styles along the processing and perceiving continuums again mapped onto Kolb's experiential learning model. By combining how the learner processes and perceives their learning, a learner is able to move through the stages of experiential learning. Again, the most effective learning is achieved through blending doing, thinking, watching and feeling. Different learning opportunities will mean you will occupy different positions on the continuum. For example, on some occasions you may be restricted to observing only, or you may choose to 'just watch' and take the opportunity to think about what you are watching. The benefit of this approach to learning is that your whole time in practice can be viewed as a learning opportunity. All the time you will be either doing something, thinking about something, watching something or feeling something.

Knowing about the different learning styles you can adopt will provide you with a focus for your learning and help you to maximise your learning in practice. Regrettably, it is still possible to attend your placement, even participate in nursing care, and still not actually experience any learning. The final section of this chapter will provide you with some

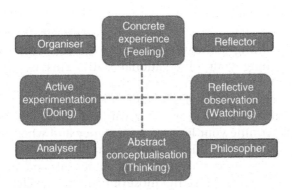

Figure 3.4 Diagram of the processing and perceiving continuums mapped onto Kolb's experiential learning cycle

guidance on how to make every experience a learning opportunity and highlight your responsibility in achieving this.

You are responsible for your own learning

The final principle of how you learn in practice is that each person owns their own learning. Your mentor and all the other professionals and practitioners that you work alongside in practice are able to facilitate and support your learning, but the extent (or lack) of your learning is ultimately your responsibility. Learning happens best when the learner is consciously engaged in constructing their knowledge, skills and attitudes. Have you been asked what you learnt in practice and it seemed hard to articulate? This suggests that perhaps you are taking too passive a role in your learning when you are in practice This section will explore the different learning strategies that you can use to maximise your learning in practice.

Strategies for learning

The learning strategies presented in this section are aligned to four types of experience that you will have in practice: exposure to an experience; participation in an experience; reflection on an experience; and reinforcement of an experience. These experiences may come about through planned activities as agreed in your learning contract or they may result from unplanned activity reflecting the real-time nature of practice that you will encounter as a student nurse.

Exposure to an experience

The primary learning strategy associated with this type of experience is about developing your observational skills. This is especially helpful when you encounter experiences that may require you to take a non-participatory role. Examples include emergency situations, the period early on in a new placement, working with a new member of staff who has as yet to determine your level of competency and when you practise a new skill (clinical or non-clinical). Other examples include observing inter-professional working, undertaking departmental visits and attending meetings or case conferences. Make the most of being in the clinical setting by accessing the experience and the expertise within the whole clinical team.

Even shadowing a practitioner, however much of an expert, does not guarantee successful learning through observing their practice alone. It is important that you agree in advance the purpose and plan for the experience. If this is not possible, and in order to avoid you going into 'screen-saver mode' when you are just observing someone or something, consider the following prompts to guide your observational skills and make the experience less passive for you:

➤ What is the patient's journey/story? – How did they get here? Where will they go after? What is their experience like?

➤ What did you notice about how, and the order in which, things were done?

➤ What would you do the same/differently in the equivalent situation?

It is also helpful to seek your own professional understanding of a situation or area of practice that you have observed. Notice the responses of others; for example, when your mentor talks with a patient what was the patient's response? By recognising both the actions and the responses to these actions you will be able to develop your practice in a more empathic and compassionate manner.

Lucy's story (Mental health nursing student)

'I needed to just watch on a number of placements as I felt too unfamiliar with the environment and the service user group. I made a point of focusing on a particular aspect such as how my mentor explained something to a service user and I would play this through in my mind and think how I would have been in the same situation. Definitely, watching is an important part of being in practice.'

As a follow-on to observing practice, you may also utilise other learning strategies such as debriefing with your mentor, leading a reflective discussion with your peers and questioning what you have observed. The observation may lead to new routes of enquiry as you conduct research into the evidence base for the practice you have observed or you may decide to review the associated policy or guidelines (local and/or national).

Participation in an experience

This is the type of experience that most students expect to have in practice; however, it is very important to not equate learning simply with doing. Research shows that students consider learning in practice is about completing a sequence or series of tasks (often associated with the completion of **activities of daily living**), and to be successful in learning is to do each task better (Ironside et al. 2014). In order to become a nurse, however, you will need to develop a more complex understanding of a service user's clinical situation and how you can contribute to their care beyond just a task-orientated approach.

Your participation in an experience is not simply about improving your motor skills or dexterity. The experience should also include learning how to interact with service users, developing your non-clinical skills and recognising the influence of **human factors**. You should aim to make sense of experiences using the following strategies:

➤ *Pattern recognition* is the process of building up the features of clinical practice by recognising these in prior experiences. An example of this is by having previously seen deterioration in service users you are more aware of the signs and symptoms of deterioration and/or you know what to do in response.

➤ *Situational awareness* is acquired through acculturation in the clinical setting while remaining cognisant of salient or critical information. An example of this is knowing the importance of identifying the service user prior to administration of a medication.

➤ *Routinised actions* is recognising which areas of practice are relevant to the individual care of a specific service user and which can be applied to the practice situation overall. An example of this is understanding the service user's condition, their preferences or expectations and the implications this has for your nursing care.

(Nadelson 2014; Fotheringham and Lamont 2015; Stacey et al. 2015)

Your learning from participation in an experience may be improved if you divide what you are intending to learn into discrete sections. This will enable you to feel less overwhelmed in your learning and give you the opportunity to test out your practice and build your confidence. Again this approach does not have to focus solely on tasks or skills acquisition; it can work equally well with developing your knowledge and attitudes. Work through Activity 3.5 to understand more about this process.

Activity 3.5 Learning from an experience in stages

Identify a learning need from an experience that you have had, for example a skill.

Deconstruct the skill; most skills are not a single skill. Instead they are a collection of skills. Examples of sub-skills include:

- writing
- researching
- building relationships
- using specific equipment
- communication skills
- knowledge of the subject

Deliberate practice – focus on specific elements of the skill that you want to learn or improve.

Discomfort zone – be aware of the aspects of the skill that require more effort for you to learn and avoid repeating elements of the skill that you are already familiar with.

Draw it together – make sure that you reconstruct your learning of the skill to be able to complete it as a whole.

Demonstrate - seek feedback from a third party as well as a self-assessment of your achievement.

Reflection on an experience

There is great benefit to learning by reflecting on your experiences in practice. Reflection involves taking a critical or evaluative stance in relation to your understanding of your own practice. It involves self-awareness of what you bring to the interactions you have with others in terms of your life experiences, values and beliefs. There are different kinds of reflection including:

➤ *Reflection on action* – this occurs after an event, either alone or in groups.

> *Reflection in action* – this is where you reflect about what you are doing and what you should do next in the moment.

> *Reflection about our impact on others* – this is where you develop your understanding of how your behaviour influences the working or therapeutic relationships you have.

> *Reflection about our own self* – this is where you increase your awareness of your strengths, weaknesses and learning needs.

Using a reflective diary can develop your skills of reflection as you record your experiences and your thoughts on these experiences. You could use a paper-based diary or the equivalent in an electronic format, or even utilise newer technologies such as video blogs (vlogs). Whichever method you choose it is important to reflect and add to your entries regularly. This process will facilitate your learning as it will support your understanding of an event or interaction, it will develop your accuracy in representing your experiences and it will develop your critical thinking skills. It will also help you to evaluate your professional behaviours in order to extract personal meaning and further learning.

Students often talk about the fear of not making as much progress as they feel they should. This might even be a topic in your diary. By reviewing past entries you will be able to see your personal and professional development and improvements in your writing and self-expression. You will be able to ascertain how, over time, you have developed your knowledge, skills and attitudes. You may note that you are more capable and that you have a more professional focus in your entries. A key time when such a review is particularly helpful is at the start of each new academic year and once you are registered and start practising as a newly qualified nurse. Appendix 8 has a list of reflective questions that can help you to start deriving meaning from your practice experiences.

Your reflective diary may be private and have an informal style. However, you will also be expected to demonstrate your skills of reflection within your academic studies and your practice documentation. Therefore, at university you will be taught about using reflective models. These are published frameworks that will guide you through a process of reflection. Gibbs' model (1988) has widely been utilised as an effective tool to aid reflection within nursing. This model adopts a cyclical approach, and if you are new to reflective thinking, it is a good starting point from which to learn the process. Figure 3.5 presents a diagram of Gibbs' reflective cycle and Activity 3.6 gets you to use this model to undertake a reflection of an event in practice.

Although it is relatively clear as to what needs to be considered at each stage of the cycle, here are some thinking points that may be helpful to gain the most from the process of reflective thinking.

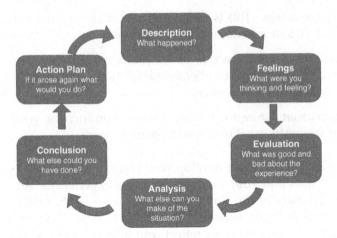

Figure 3.5   The reflective cycle (Gibbs 1988)

The reflective learning cycle was originally published in G. Gibbs (1988) *Learning by Doing: A Guide to Teaching and Learning Methods*. Further Education Unit. Oxford Polytechnic: Oxford. This book is now available to download as an ebook from the website of the Oxford Centre for Staff and Learning Development, Oxford Brookes University at http://www.brookes.ac.uk/ocsld/publications/

Activity 3.6

Utilising the model of reflection proposed by Gibbs (see Figure 3.5), consider a recent event or incident you were involved in and follow the cycle to undertake a reflection.

What was using the process like?

Did you think more about the event as a result of using the model?

Have you identified any new learning needs?

Did you decide to write down this reflection or talk it through with someone else?

Description

This is the starting point within the process, and is the time for you to outline what it is you are reflecting upon. This may be a new learning experience, an incident from practice or indeed anything that has got you thinking and looking to make sense of a situation. It is helpful to outline some background information and some rationale as to why you are reflecting on this particular issue. Set the scene in terms of who was involved (remembering confidentiality!) and outline any other important details such as time of day, placement type and so on. Do remember that unless you are using this cycle to support academic writing there is no word limit for personal use, so although you may wish to be precise and to the point you can add as much information as you see fit. This will be of benefit in weeks, months and years to come when you reread your reflections, as it will remind you of how you were feeling at the time and of all the key details.

Feelings

In this section document exactly how you were feeling at the time of the event. For obvious reasons reflection ideally needs to take place as close to the actual event as possible, as the more time there is between the event and when the reflective thinking occurs, the less you will be able to accurately recollect your feelings. You can ask yourself a number of direct questions to help with this section:

➤ What was I feeling at the time?

➤ What was I thinking at the time?

➤ What did I do at the time?

➤ What were other people doing at the time and how did I feel about those actions?

As these are your own personal thoughts do feel empowered to be as open and honest with yourself as possible.

Evaluation

This section enables you to consider in detail how well you think the experience was managed at the time, and allows you to think about how you acted or dealt with the situation you found yourself in. If the reflection relates to an upsetting or challenging incident, what are your thoughts in relation to the overall way in which it was managed? Why do you feel this way? Ensure that you think about both the positive and what you may consider to be negative aspects of the experience. Hopefully you will soon see that what you originally perceived as negative can be viewed as key areas for learning and further reflection.

Analysis

This section is the key part in which to try and make sense of what has occurred. Can you relate it to any literature or documented theory that you have read previously? If not, it may be a good time to look into what has already been written on the experience. Is there anything that states how such an event should have been managed?

Conclusion

Having utilised the earlier stages of the cycle, what are your thoughts now? Is there anything that you feel you could have done differently? Was there another approach to dealing with the event that may have had a different outcome? If the event was positive, would any other actions or behaviours have led to the same identical outcome?

Action plan

This final stage is just as important as the first stage of the cycle, as it gives you the opportunity to sum everything up in order to set your learning needs. For instance, do you feel that training is required to ensure that if the event was to repeat itself you would be better prepared? If this is the case, how will you ensure this training is delivered? If you feel a greater level of knowledge or understanding is required ensure that you take the time to meet with your allocated mentor to discuss the event. You may or may not wish to ask them to read your reflective account to assist with this process. If your mentor is not the most appropriate person to talk to, ensure that you seek out support from within the university, as the important component of reflective thinking is that you don't just reflect, leave it alone and then repeat exactly the same set of actions. The whole point of reflection is to learn, build new knowledge and skills and move forward, hence the fact that this is often viewed as a cyclical process.

An alternative to Gibbs' reflective cycle is Johns' model (1994) for structured reflection. This is also cyclical and is reproduced in Figure 3.6 followed by a breakdown of what to do in each stage.

As you can see, the model is based upon a five-stage approach, a number of which are similar to the six stages of Gibbs' reflective cycle.

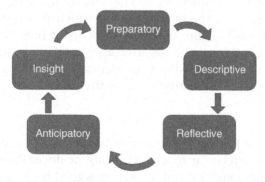

Figure 3.6 Adaption of Johns' model (2013) for structured reflection into a learning cycle

Preparatory

The initial stage of reflection is becoming mindful of the experience by drawing on the emotional, cognitive and physical qualities and characteristics of the experience.

Descriptive

The process continues by outlining the key circumstances relating to the event itself, including what you feel to be the most significant factors. The description should be of sufficient detail that someone not involved in the event can gain a clear understanding of what occurred.

Reflective

Give thought to what you were trying to achieve, and what were the consequences, if any, of the event? You need to consider if there were any factors that influenced your actions and behaviours resulting from your lack of knowledge or experience. While reflecting do bear in mind that the journey to become a nurse is a complex one, and you will be exposed to many situations that highlight gaps in your knowledge and understanding. But having identified these deficits you will then be able to address them.

Anticipatory

This stage of the model encourages you to consider if there were any other ways of managing the event and, if so, whether the outcome could have been different in any way. Your reflection can focus on positive events, as well as those that are more challenging. It is helpful to consider what you did well and how to repeat this as much as what you could improve upon.

Insight

This final stage is very similar to the action plan element of Gibbs' cycle, as it requires you to think about what you have learnt and what insights you have gained in order to determine what needs to happen now – What learning do you need to initiate? Will you change your practice in any way? Will you need to seek out support to build your knowledge or skill base?

Reinforcement of an experience

In order to reinforce your learning from experiences you should make use of the following learning strategies:

➤ questioning

➤ repeating practice

➤ teaching others.

Questioning is a helpful means of reinforcing what you have learnt. On the one hand you will answer questions asked by your mentor, a service user, your colleagues or your peers, and on the other you will ask them questions. There are two broad types of questions with differing purposes:

➤ Closed questions – where there is a fixed response to the question. These types of questions are best used for memory recall or checking comprehension of factual information; for example, what are the normal ranges of the basic observations?

➤ Open questions – where there is no fixed response to the question. These types of questions are best used for the application of knowledge to new/novel situations, to identify the rationale for your actions/ interactions and to provide strategies for gaining understanding and meaning from experiences; for example, in which situations would you check someone's basic observations? How will you troubleshoot if you are unable to measure someone's basic observations? What do you understand was happening when we were taking the patient's observations?

Your mentor will want you to be able to learn, and to feel comfortable in asking questions. After all, no matter where you are on placement or what you are doing, if you do not know something you will need to ask. It is perfectly acceptable to ask questions – in fact, your mentor will be expecting them! On occasions, it may not be appropriate to ask a question at the time, particularly if direct care is being given. You may find that carrying a small notebook or using your phone is useful to note down thoughts and questions in order that you ask them later in the shift.

When asking questions try to avoid the common trap of directing 'why' questions towards the person. Why says defend or justify. Therefore, rather than 'Why did you do that?' try as an alternative, 'What were you wanting to achieve by doing it in that way?' or 'What stopped you following policy?' You will hopefully get a less defensive response and you will appear less accusatory.

Repeating practice is a common method for reinforcing learning. Through repetition your knowledge, skills and attitudes will be tested and strengthened. This strategy can be linked to assessment, for example you may undertake several formative assessments before completing a summative assessment (see Chapter 6 – 'When?' – for more information on assessment). Alternatively, you will have the opportunity to try out clinical skills and simulation taught at university within the CLE. This is helpful as you will be better prepared for your time in practice and able to focus only on the elements of the skill that you need to rehearse.

It is more than likely that you will encounter repeated situations in practice; certain activities are routine and will recur on a weekly, daily or even hourly basis. Your participation in these activities will vary according to your level of competence and familiarity, but often with repetition you will be able to refine and improve your knowledge, skills and attitudes.

Teaching others is a great way to reinforce your learning. Your experience of teaching does not have to be formal, even simply conveying information to another person will enable you to gauge your level of understanding and your ability to present concepts and ideas in a coherent manner. Teaching is similar to the technique of questioning in that you can direct your teaching to the same people. In fact, you may start to teach as a way of answering a person's question. When you teach consider the following elements:

> ➤ What does the person want to learn?

> ➤ What do I know about the subject?

> ➤ Do I need to learn anything else?

> ➤ What is the best way to teach this?

> ➤ How do I know that the person has learnt it?

The above learning strategies are not intended to be a definitive list. Instead they will hopefully act as a springboard and help you to maintain responsibility for your learning. It is your choice how you learn: do you want to observe or participate in an experience? How will you reflect on this experience and what is the best way to reinforce your learning in future practice experiences?

Summary

This chapter has looked in detail at the principles of how you learn in practice. The first principle is that you have the ability to learn. This is subject to your level of motivation which is based on external and internal drivers, such as receiving clear instructions and having a sense of achievement. Having established your readiness to learn you will also need to display the right attributes of a learner. During your time in practice you will need to learn how to integrate, transition, assimilate and progress your knowledge, skills and attitudes.

Despite having knowledge of how you learn you will meet challenges to your learning. These may be situational – for example, your unfamiliarity with the placement – or dependent on your ability to manage issues in practice – for example, your response to stress. By fostering the intrinsic qualities of a learner, such as communication, questioning skills and critical thinking, and being emotionally intelligent you will be better able to overcome such issues in practice.

It is important to recognise that there is support available to you. In view of the challenges to your learning that you may face you should have a low threshold for seeking help so that your time on placement is directed towards learning rather than just coping or feeling overwhelmed. You will receive support from staff in practice and at university; the extrinsic requirements that you should expect your mentor and other people in the CLE to provide have been described. As well as receiving support you have access to support mechanisms to help you build your resilience and manage your anxiety. If you have a specific learning requirement you should also be supported in practice with a learning support plan detailing the reasonable adjustments that need to be made to best facilitate your learning.

The second principle is that you learn in different ways. The advantage of acknowledging how you learn means that you can make improvements to your learning and you can adjust your learning style to fit the learning opportunity. Three groups of learning styles were presented: the Honey and Mumford learning styles – activist, theorist, pragmatist and reflector; the 'modes of learning' – visual, aural, read/write and kinaesthetic; and the 'processing and perceiving continuum' – analyser, organiser, philosopher and reflector. You were encouraged to identify your learning style by completing the Honey and Mumford Learning Styles Questionnaire. Each learning style has an associated range of preferred learning and teaching activities, and the learning styles were mapped against Kolb's experiential learning cycle to demonstrate that learning is best achieved when a combination of learning styles are used and the learner uses a modifiable approach to their learning.

The final principle of how you learn is that you are responsible for your learning. This involves employing various strategies for learning, from exposure to, participation in, reflection on and reinforcement of your learning experiences. Developing your skills of observation, questioning and reflection will enhance your learning in practice and ensure that every experience you encounter can be a source of learning.

Knowledge review

See Appendix 3 to compare your answers.

1. What examples can you give of building up your resilience?

2. What are the benefits to you knowing your learning style?

3. What are the four learning styles and how are they defined according to Honey and Mumford?

4. What are the four broad learning strategies?

Further reading and resources

Honey and Mumford Learning Styles: http://www.brainboxx.co.uk/
    a2_learnstyles/pages/learningstyles.htm
Visual, Aural, Read/Write, Kinaesthetic: http://vark-learn.com/
Kolb's Learning Styles Inventory: http://www.lifecircles-inc.com/
    Learningtheories/constructivism/kolb.html
Learning to Learn: http://www.nwlink.com/~donclark/hrd/styles/learn_style_
    survey.html
Royal College of Nursing Guidance for Mentors: https://www.uclan.
    ac.uk/students/study/schools/school_of_health/plsu/files/health_plsu_
    rcnmentorguidance.pdf
Boingboing Resilience Website: http://www.boingboing.org.uk/
Reflective Models: http://www.brainboxx.co.uk/a3_aspects/pages/
    ReflectionModels.htm

4

What?

Learning outcomes

After reading and completing the activities in this chapter you will be able to:

➤ Define the purpose of the Assessment of Practice document.

➤ Explore how to use the Assessment of Practice document.

➤ Examine the knowledge, skills and attitudes required of a nurse.

Your nursing course has been validated against the Nursing and Midwifery Council (NMC) standards for pre-registration nursing education (NMC 2010) which specifies what you need to learn to be assessed as competent. The hallmark of your registration is that you possess the knowledge, skills and attitudes to practise safely and effectively. Being in practice will mean organising and prioritising your learning so that you are able to learn fully how to reason as a nurse (knowledge), how to perform as a nurse (skills) and how to act as a nurse (attitudes).

The evidence on the preparedness of graduate nurses suggests many newly registered nurses feel underprepared. The transition to qualified practitioner can be overwhelming, with high levels of reported stress as a response to facing the realities of the clinical setting (Purling and King 2012). Particular areas of concern for graduate nurses were their lack of knowledge in problem solving and clinical decision making (Etheridge 2007; Purling and King 2012; Esmaeili et al. 2014). Furthermore, a study by Bagnardi (2014) identified that graduate nurses were not practising at the level required in several other areas including delegation, risk assessment, conflict resolution and clinical prioritisation. Alongside the gaps in their learning, graduates have also reported their immersion into clinical practice was too rapid, in spite of a **preceptorship** period, as they faced a major change in the role when transitioning from student to nurse (Watt and Pascoe 2013). The change in role comprises not only learning how to be an employee and a member of a team but also accepting the account-ability of being a nurse and acting as an autonomous professional (Bull et al. 2015).

Coupled with these challenges of preparedness and change of role are the demands of contemporary healthcare that will increasingly mean nurses will be caring for people with complex health and social care needs and co-morbidities. Therefore, the knowledge, skills and attitudes you will be required to learn should prepare you to practise with confidence, to transition seamlessly into a registered nurse and to anticipate and manage the care needs of service users. The three years of your course are therefore vital to allow you sufficient exposure to experiences, time to process infor-mation and opportunities to synthesise this learning into your practice.

This chapter examines what you need to learn to become a nurse. It is subdivided into sections that highlight the significant knowledge, skills and attitudes that you will be engaged in learning while in practice. Cap-turing what you have learnt is a necessary part of being a student nurse. Therefore, this chapter will begin with an exploration of the Assessment of Practice document.

Assessment of Practice (AOP) document

You will have an Assessment of Practice (AOP) document to complete during your time on placement. You may know it by another name, for example practice assessment document (PAD), practice portfolio, ongoing record of achievement (ORA) or it may simply be referred to as the 'skills book' (a common misnomer). The AOP document may be in hard copy or electronic form and you may receive a single document to be completed over the duration of the whole course or separate documents to be com-pleted every year. The AOP document is your evidence of achieving the required competencies and skills. Therefore, your primary responsibility is to keep the document safe. You will also be responsible for ensuring that you and your **mentor** complete the document accurately. Activity 4.1 will help you become more effective in using the document.

The first thing to note about the document is although its title focuses on evidencing your learning through assessment, the document will also have been designed to facilitate your learning and preparation for assess-ment. Consequently, the following sections will often be included in the document:

➢ learning contracts (more information given in this section)

➢ learning activity logs

Activity 4.1 Assessment of Practice document

- How well do you understand the document?
- How do you use the document to guide your learning and assessment?
- What questions do you have about the document?
- What is useful/not useful about the document?

These questions would also be helpful to put to your mentor so that they too can use the document effectively.

➤ feedback reports

➤ reflective accounts

➤ formative assessments

➤ action plans (more information given in this section).

A **learning contract** is an individualised agreement between you and your mentor of your learning needs (Bailey and Tuohy 2009). The use of a learning contract helps to focus your learning by recording your specific learning needs and the process by which your learning will be achieved. Setting a learning contract will tend to increase your contact time with your mentor as you will have something to refer back to as you review your progress on placement. The development of a learning contract involves following key stages (see Figure 4.1).

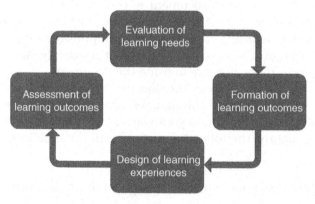

Figure 4.1   Diagram of the stages of developing a learning contract

The evaluation of your learning needs is about identifying the gap between your current knowledge, skills and attitudes and the level of knowledge, skills and attitudes required. This self-assessment could take the form of:

➤ a 'Strengths, Weaknesses, Opportunities and Threats' (SWOT) analysis (see Appendix 9)

➤ a reflection on your previous experiences, your achievements and the areas of your knowledge, skills and attitudes that you need to improve

➤ a review of your progress towards achieving the NMC competencies and fulfilling the four NMC domains: professional values; communication and interpersonal skills; nursing practice and decision making; and leadership, management and team working.

Please note that the sum total of your learning needs should not just be a list of the remaining skills you need to complete in the AOP document. You should challenge yourself when you simply use placements as the means to get skills signed off. Your learning in practice will often be more meaningful if you immerse yourself in the clinical learning environment (CLE) and establish learning needs that could otherwise be missed. For example, you may have the need to learn how to develop a deeper understanding of a clinical specialty or how to transfer your prior knowledge and skills into a new clinical area.

Emmanuel's story (Mental Health nursing student)

'Now I am in my second year I want to get more out of placements. It is always a balance between what I have to achieve and get recorded in my book and what I could learn in each placement. Whilst I like the freedom of choosing my own learning I sometimes don't see the 'wood for the trees' and my mentor says 'You don't need to know that, better to focus on this instead' which I appreciate.'

Jarek's story (Learning Disabilities nursing student)

'When I meet each mentor I say 'I want to be like you. Can you teach me how?' Most just laugh but that is basically what I need.'

Having completed your self-assessment and identified your learning needs, using this information you and your mentor will formulate your learning outcomes. Learning outcomes are a descriptive statement of what you will be able to do following a period of learning. Learning outcomes should be specific and achievable within the time frame and the context of the placement. It is helpful to assign dates for when each of the learning outcomes should be achieved. Some may require the full length of the placement in order to be achieved, whereas others can be achieved in a relatively short space of time.

The following are examples of learning outcomes from student learning contracts:

➤ Develop an understanding of therapeutic relationships throughout the placement and gather evidence for NMC domain 2: communication and interpersonal skills.

➤ Perform a variety of nursing roles (advocate, educator, manager, researcher) – that is, managerial roles. Work with the shift leader, team leader and nurse manager and in the final two weeks of the placement complete the nursing management skill.

➤ Gain experience of service user admission/discharge within the first week of the placement and undertake an indirectly supervised admission/discharge by week 6 of the placement.

➤ Develop skills in physical/psychological assessment of patients. Complete a documented assessment and handover of findings to senior staff each week and if possible include in this an assessment of a deteriorating patient.

➤ Contribute to the assessment, planning, implementation and evaluation of nursing care for a group of service users for NMC domain 3: nursing practice and decision making by week 8 of the placement.

➤ Create and utilise opportunities to promote the health and well-being of service users in each clinic appointment and seek service user feedback on their experience.

➤ Apply research evidence to clinical practice by undertaking a literature review of pain management in infants and discussing findings with mentor by week 6 of the placement.

➤ Utilise clinical frameworks and risk assessment tools for service user assessment and nursing care and be observed by mentor, completing a risk assessment in the final week of placement.

Following the creation of your learning outcomes you and your mentor will need to design your learning experiences. These will be planned in order to help you meet your learning outcomes and accommodate your learning support plan (see Chapter 3 – 'How?'). The experiences should be relevant and assigned according to your level of competency and the level of mentor supervision required. The learning opportunities should identify which service users and activities you can be involved with. Your mentor should be fully involved in developing your learning experiences because of their knowledge of the resources and the range of learning opportunities available to you in the specific placement.

The final stage of the learning contract is assessment of the learning outcomes. A learning contract can give you a real sense of accomplishment as you complete your learning outcomes and measure the extent of your learning. Therefore, the learning contract should also include how each learning outcome will be assessed. Examples of assessment include observing your practice, receiving service user feedback and reviewing your evidence of achieving the NMC competencies. Chapter 6 – 'When?' – provides more details on assessment for learning.

Action plans are a means of feeding forward your learning in to your next placement. Whereas a learning contract is speculative, that is, it contains what you hope to learn/achieve in the placement, an action plan is definitive. It will contain precise learning needs that may be outstanding from the learning contract or identified subsequently in the placement, for example as a result of failing a skill or only partially completing an NMC competency. The SMART model – that is, actions need to be Specific, Measureable, Achievable, Realistic and achieved within a Timescale – is recommended to be used as the basis of your action plan. The action plan devised in partnership with your mentor should avoid broad statements such as, 'Needs to improve communication'. A more specific action would be defining the type of communication that needs to be improved – for example, does your verbal communication need to be improved and if so with whom, or do you need to develop your written communication? Having clear and unambiguous actions makes them more achievable. See Table 4.1 for a template action plan based on the SMART model.

The AOP document also functions as a means of recording where your learning takes place. You will be required to record details of each placement that you attend, including the title of the clinical area, the type of placement and the name of your mentor. Chapter 2 – 'Where?' – discusses the variety of placements that exist to enable you to gain exposure to a range of health and social care settings. Due to the individual nature of

Table 4.1 Action plan (template)

Specific action	What action are you wanting to achieve?
	What are the steps to achieving it?
Measureable	How will you and others know when you have achieved this action?
Achievable	What is needed to achieve this action, i.e. resources?
	Who is needed to help you achieve this action?
Realistic	How does achieving this action help in developing your knowledge, skills and attitude for becoming a nurse?
Timescale	When do you intend, and will you need, to review your progress to achieving this action?

your learning needs, your learning experiences will not be the same as another student who has attended or currently is attending the same placement. Having said that, if you discuss your placement with your colleagues, you may gain helpful insights into the placement in terms of what learning opportunities are available. There is a risk that the colleague may have nothing positive to say but it is best to reserve judgement and use the appropriate feedback/evaluation mechanisms if you do have any concerns. It is possible that improvements could be made to the placement to make it a model CLE. Chapter 2 – 'Where?' – also explores this.

If nurses are present in a placement and working (safely and effectively) you will have the opportunity to learn. You may not be particularly interested in the speciality or clinical area (which would be helpful to discuss with your mentor) but there will always be opportunities to develop your knowledge, to enhance your skills and to improve your professional attitude. You could direct your learning towards a general concept of nursing practice – for example, communication – and see how this applies in the particular placement. You may choose to focus on the service user experience and assess the impact of the care they are receiving on them and their family. You will even find by simply participating in the day-to-day activity of the placement that you can learn to understand routines and the rationales for practice.

The next three sections of this chapter go through in more detail the associated knowledge, skills and attitudes of a registered nurse, focusing on areas that are considered more difficult to acquire or reportedly lacking at the point of registration. It is not feasible to provide an exhaustive list of what you need to learn as this would soon become out of date owing to the rapid pace of change in clinical practice. Please refer to Chapter 1 – 'Why?' – for the competencies and skills scheduled in the

NMC **competency framework** and the **essential skills clusters** (ESC) that are required for entry to the register.

It is important to note that the sections are not written in order of priority, that is, knowledge is of no greater or lesser importance than skills or attitudes. Similarly, for ease of presentation the three areas have been separated out. However, in practice your knowledge, skills and attitudes cannot be isolated. Being a registered nurse requires demonstration of all three areas for your practice to be safe and effective; and it is also entirely possible to be knowledgeable and skilled but lacking a professional attitude. This would not be considered as safe and effective practice. Ultimately practice is the place where you can draw together your learning and demonstrate your competence as a professional with the right knowledge, skills and attitudes as a whole.

Knowledge

Nursing knowledge provides the evidence base for your practice. The term **evidence-based practice** (EBP) refers to the integration of the clinician's knowledge with the best available research evidence, guided by professional values in the process of making decisions for the care of service users. In essence, it is working in a way that is known to be the safest and the most effective way of doing so.

Types of knowledge

There are different forms of knowledge that the nurse will use to inform their EBP: propositional and practical (tacit) knowledge.

Propositional knowledge

During your nursing course you will learn much propositional knowledge, partly because it is the most frequently taught knowledge type, but also because it encompasses learning facts, statements and rules. In the care of people there is no margin of error and therefore it is essential to have absolute knowledge about human anatomy and physiology, pathophysiology, how medications work, how to use a medical device and how to work out a drug calculation. Try Activity 4.2 to see if you can add to this list.

Activity 4.2 Examples of propositional knowledge

What other fact-based examples of nursing knowledge can you list?

What was the source of this knowledge?

- a lecture?

- your mentor?

- a colleague?

- independent study?

- the internet?

Did you just accept this knowledge or did you verify it; and, if so, how?

How have you applied this knowledge in your practice?

This type of knowledge can be difficult to learn, it often assumes a prior level of knowledge or understanding which you may not have (e.g. chemistry). You may have to acquire a new language (e.g. medical terminology) to even access this knowledge and it may bring back negative associations of earlier educational experiences (e.g. calculations and mathematics). Propositional knowledge is often considered definitive but new information is continually emerging which overrides or supersedes previously accepted knowledge, for example what is considered to be a mental disorder now is very different from previous classifications and diagnoses. There are issues surrounding the validity of this knowledge, for example the falsification of data or poor research methodologies may reduce its trustworthiness. And there are issues surrounding the applicability of this knowledge, for example you may have understood everything there is to know about cellular signalling but this bears no relevance to the more immediate need of knowing how to communicate with a person who is confused and agitated. The limitations of propositional knowledge mean that other knowledge types are equally necessary. In particular, the latter limitation of propositional knowledge suggests that having practical knowledge will greatly benefit your practice.

Practical knowledge

Practical knowledge encompasses that which is learnt through experiences, such as the performance of skills. The development of expertise or intuition is acquired through practical knowledge which involves familiarity and repetition. Practical knowledge can also be understood as tacit knowledge whereby knowledge is communicated through consistent contact with an expert (such as your mentor or a service user). This knowledge is gained through informal means that is often difficult to write down or transfer from one individual to another. Such knowledge can be conveyed through body language, humour, or the ease and confidence displayed by your mentor in their practice. There will be occasions when formal teaching is arranged for you, maybe in advance of a skill-based assessment. Yet simply being in the CLE means your exposure to tacit knowledge is occurring all the time. For example, by observing interactions between staff and service users you will pick up cues of how to respond, you will foster complex social skills by participating in teamwork and you will develop an aesthetic sense of nursing through immersion in practice.

Using your practical (tacit) knowledge will involve some propositional knowledge as well. For example, if you know practically how to administer a subcutaneous injection then you presumably know some facts (propositional knowledge) about aseptic non-touch technique, the sites of injection and so on. This illustration exemplifies the relationship between learning and knowledge. Learning is the means to accumulate knowledge. However, simply amassing knowledge is neither appropriate nor feasible for your nursing education. To guide what you need to know and therefore learn you need to use a theory. Before working through what theory is used in nursing, it may be helpful for you to explore your own understanding of theory as a term in Activity 4.3.

Activity 4.3 What is your understanding of theory?

- How would you describe what 'theory' is?

- What are your thoughts on learning theory?

  o Positive

  o Negative

- What does it mean to apply theory to practice?

- Can you think of an example when you have applied theory to your practice? What happened?

- Can you think of an example when you have not applied theory to your practice? What happened?

Nursing is an intellectual discipline; it is not just the carrying out of clinical tasks. Therefore, theory is the means for you to think. It will help you explain and understand what you experience, what you observe, what you know and what you can do. During your course you will study a number of '-ologies' such as psychology, sociology, pharmacology, physiology, pathophysiology and so on. These are specific fields of study with specialist knowledge and practice. This is one of the great aspects of nursing theory: that nurses assimilate knowledge from many different sources and apply it to their practice.

Applying knowledge to practice should not be considered as a one-way approach where knowledge governs practice. Rather knowledge and practice are interrelated in as much as knowledge guides practice; likewise practice is a means of determining knowledge deficits. What in practice is still poorly understood? This will act as the catalyst for further research and the development of new knowledge.

There is a tendency to either overemphasise or dismiss the role of theory in nursing. However, theory is a necessary part of any profession, as it provides a framework on which the principles of the profession are built. And it validates the purposes and activities of the professional. Put simply, theory defines what nursing is and what a nurse does. This is very important to establish and make known, as without it the role of the nurse is subject to unfounded changes. This does not mean that nursing must remain the same. Clearly, advances in healthcare and increasing demand on services will mean that nurses must respond to and meet these challenges. But by understanding the scope and boundaries of nursing, the manner in which this change occurs should remain true to the core values and practices of nursing.

Nursing is understood within a framework of four metaparadigms (yes, the use of big words is the most common criticism of theory!). A metaparadigm is basically the overarching view of a profession or discipline. It identifies what concepts are of interest to the discipline and the relationships that exist between these concepts. The agreed theory of nursing is based on Lee and Fawcett's work in 1978, which defined four metaparadigms central to nursing, namely the human being, nursing, health and the environment (Lee and Fawcett 2013). It is anticipated that you have been or will be taught about this at some point on your course. Figure 4.2 illustrates that the human being should remain at the centre of nursing theory.

It is important to remember that understanding nursing theory is not an abstract task but a necessary and meaningful activity. For example, the practice of assessing a service user is based on the following theoretical underpinning: nurses assess, nursing is directed towards a person and nurses communicate what they do. The knowledge required to achieve

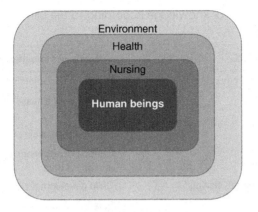

Figure 4.2 Diagram of the four nursing metaparadigms

this in practice includes understanding how to conduct a physical/ psychological assessment, knowing how to establish a therapeutic relationship and having an awareness of completing accurate records and communicating assessment findings.

Developing knowledge

It can be helpful to your learning to determine the specific knowledge that could be gained from each CLE (see the examples provided in Table 4.2).

Areas of knowledge that students report as difficult to learn include the following.

Risk assessment

Nurses are central in the assessment of risk for service users. Risk assessment is about ascertaining risk and the ways in which risk can be minimised. The principles of risk assessment are to first identify the hazard – the thing that will cause harm – and then work out the risk, that is, the likelihood of the hazard happening, and the severity of harm that could result. Take a common hazard – falling; from this you could learn about the mechanism of falling, the impact of falls on the individual and the health service, the prevalence of falls, who is at risk of falls, the methods of falls prevention and what to do in the event of a fall. As you can see, risk assessment is an ideal means of stimulating and broadening your knowledge.

Table 4.2 Examples of knowledge according to the clinical learning environment (CLE)

Clinical setting	CLE	Examples of specific knowledge
Community	Community nursing	Public and population health
		Chronicity of disease/mental health disorder
		Hospital admission prevention
		Context of community nursing in health and social care
	Health visiting	Child development
		Safeguarding
		Family work
	Child and adolescent mental health services	Child development
		Safeguarding
		Family work
		Childhood mental health disorders
Acute	Critical care/Emergency department	Trauma, burns
		Advanced clinical practice
		Triage
		Suicide prevention
	In-patient mental health	Mental health specialties
		Mental health disorders
		Acute presentation
		24/7 care
		Mental health techniques and treatments
		Rehabilitation
		Context of acute nursing in health and social care
	Surgical	Surgical specialties
		Surgical pathologies
		Acute presentations
		24/7 care
		Surgical techniques/treatments
		Pre-, peri- and post-operative care
		Rehabilitation
		Context of acute nursing in health and social care

Medical	Medical specialties
	Medical pathologies
	Acute presentations
	24/7 care
	Medical techniques/treatments
	Rehabilitation
	Context of acute nursing in health and social care

It is hoped that by becoming vigilant to the potential harm caused by healthcare (in general) and in your own practice (in particular) you will learn how to avoid harm and manage risks. Activity 4.4 will help you develop your awareness of hazards for service users.

Activity 4.4 What hazards are your service users exposed to?

A hazard is something with the potential to cause harm or have an adverse effect on health. Remember this may not just be a physical effect, as certain hazards will also cause psychological harm.

Answer the following questions to identify hazards in your placement.

- Review the activities of the clinical area:

  o Who is performing these activities? (registered or unregistered, trained or untrained)

  o Which activities involve the service user directly?

  o What activities are routine or non-routine?

  o When are these activities carried out? (day- or night-time)

- Look at accident/incident/near-miss records – what harm or near misses have service users been subject to?

- What equipment is in use in the clinical area?

- Consider groups of people that may have a different level of risk such as inexperienced staff, persons with disabilities, persons who are confused.

- What hazards could visitors be exposed to?

Now consider whether the hazard can be eliminated or only controlled.

Certain risks that are deemed preventable have already been identified in specific populations. As a result assessment tools or scales (often more than one) have been produced for healthcare professionals to use to screen for the individual's risk and their risk factors. Using this information the healthcare professional can provide care to avoid or further reduce the risk.

Examples of risk assessment tools include:

➤ *Assessment of Interpersonal Risk*, for people with learning disabilities who have challenging behaviour.

➤ *Lester Tool*, for assessing the cardiac and metabolic health of people with mental illnesses.

➤ *Malnutrition Universal Screening Tool*, to assess risk of malnutrition for any adult (an equivalent is available for children – *Screening Tool for the Assessment of Malnutrition in Paediatrics*).

➤ *Paediatric Observation Priority Score*, a system to detect serious illness in children.

➤ *Purpose T*, for the assessment of pressure damage and pressure ulcer formation in adults.

➤ *Suicide Risk Assessment Tool*, for screening for self-harm and suicide risk in any population.

➤ *Venous Thromboembolism (VTE) Risk Assessment*, to assess risk of VTE formation in any population.

While these tools can be helpful they are only valid if used correctly. Your role when in practice is to learn how to complete the assessment tools accurately. This will mean ensuring the following:

➤ Do you understand the purpose of the tool?

➤ What is the hazard and the risk (likelihood and severity of harm) being assessed?

➤ Do you understand the terminology used in the tool?

➤ Is it clear to you how to complete the tool?

➤ How do you acquire the information necessary to complete the assessment? For example, do you need to know certain facts about the service user, such as their height, their smoking history, their past medical history and so on?

➢ How do you document your answers?

➢ Once you have completed the assessment what do you do with this information?

➢ When do you reassess?

➢ Even if the service user is deemed low risk how do you keep them at this level?

Developing your risk assessment knowledge involves recognising hazards, exploring the effect of the hazard and understanding the likelihood and severity of harm. Your knowledge should also encompass a thorough understanding of extant risk assessment tools.

Clinical decision making

Despite clinical decision making being a routine activity for a nurse, the knowledge of how to make clinical decisions appears to remain somewhat of a mystery to many students. As the decisions you make will affect service users, it is integral to attain this knowledge in order to provide safe and effective care. It is helpful to consider this knowledge as being made up of stages, that is, in order to make a clinical decision you first need to know how to:

➢ Assess and interpret data/findings – Stages 1 and 2

➢ Think critically – Stage 3

➢ Problem solve – Stage 4

➢ Prioritise – Stage 5

➢ Make the clinical decision – Stage 6

By developing your knowledge in each stage of the clinical decision making process you should be better able to make sound clinical decisions. The cognitive processes needed to develop this knowledge can be classified according to the Revision of Bloom's Taxonomy by Krathwohl and colleagues (2013). The Revision of Bloom's Taxonomy is formed by two dimensions. The first dimension, identified as 'the knowledge dimension', determines the kind of knowledge to be learnt, while the second, identified as 'the cognitive process dimension', categorises the processes used to learn this knowledge. Applying the Revised Bloom's Taxonomy to clinical decision making is presented in Table 4.3:

Table 4.3 Bloom's Taxonomy as applied to clinical decision making

The stages of clinical decision making	Cognitive process	Knowledge
Assess data/findings	Remembering	Recall how to conduct an assessment, e.g. physical assessment, admission assessment, ongoing monitoring, pain assessment, responding to change in service user health/well-being and so on.
Interpret data/findings	Understanding	Summarise the information gained from the assessment and interpret it against norms or an accepted standard, e.g. normal ranges, stages of a disease, a policy/guideline and so on.
Problem solving	Applying	Classify the findings into areas of concern (actual and potential), e.g. increased confusion, reduced appetite, increased pain, pressure ulcer formation, and so on.
Critical thinking	Analysing	Determine how the findings and the problems relate to one another, e.g. what problems is the high temperature causing and why has this temperature arisen?
Prioritising	Evaluating	Rank the problems in order of priority based on criteria and standards, e.g. algorithms, guidelines, local practice, and so on.
Clinical decision making	Creating	Put together all the elements of the process to construct the decision, e.g. make a referral, continue to monitor, explain the situation to the service user, and so on. Once actualised be prepared to return to Stage 1: assess data and findings to generate a new decision.

Delegation

Knowing how to make clinical decisions is important but equally important is for the nurse to know who should carry out the decision. Delegation is another area that student nurses often report as difficult to learn.

Akram's story (Adult nursing student)

'I was always so busy on my shifts. I understood what needed to be done and then other things would crop up and I just kept going. I was often told by mentors I was doing such a good job and so I learnt that this was the right way to work. But it was a healthcare assistant on a placement who said: 'You need to ask me to help you sometimes. We are a team, it's not just down to you."

The value of delegation is that it will unburden you from unnecessary work that others are capable of completing. You need to accept that the care of a service user cannot be carried out by you (the nurse) alone. The issue of delegation is often related to a lack of understanding about accountability. Registered nurses are legally accountable for their practice, including any delegated task. Section 11 of The Code (NMC 2015) states the nurse is accountable for his/her decision to delegate tasks and duties to other people. To achieve this you must:

> 11.1 only delegate tasks and duties that are within the other person's scope of competence, making sure that they fully understand your instructions

> 11.2 make sure that everyone you delegate tasks to is adequately supervised and supported so they can provide safe and compassionate care, and

> 11.3 confirm that the outcome of any task you have delegated to someone else meets the required standard.

Some of the tasks typically delegated, for example turning, ambulating, providing personal care and blood glucose checking, are directly associated with nurse-sensitive outcomes, such as preventing complications and maintaining physiologic balance. Therefore, in order to comply with The Code and nursing targets you need to be able to answer the following questions:

How do you know the task is appropriate to delegate?

➢ Check the task is necessary

➢ Check delegation is in the patient's best interest

➢ Check the person accepts responsibility for the task.

How do you know the person has the ability to perform the task?

➢ Ask the person directly

➢ Check their job description

➢ Check local policy

➢ Observe them carry out the task.

How do you know the task has been completed satisfactorily?

➢ Communicate the objectives and goals of the task

➢ Explain the expectations of the person and the delegated task

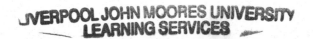

➤ Agree upon a time frame to complete the task

➤ Make sure the person knows they can check in with you/ask questions if they are unsure.

As a student you will need to learn the answers to these questions. However, you should be mindful of the following:

➤ As a student you are not accountable for your own practice, therefore any delegation that you make should be under your mentor's supervision who is accountable for your care.

➤ You may not know fully how to complete the task yourself and would therefore be unable to anticipate the full extent of the delegation.

➤ You may not feel at ease in the team to delegate.

➤ You may not have the communication skills to communicate what needs to be done.

Conflict resolution

The final area of knowledge that students are reluctant to learn about is conflict resolution. In certain clinical specialties you will receive **conflict resolution training** to manage challenging behaviour. On these courses you will learn skills and techniques to help you break away and protect yourself when threatened or physically assaulted. Your likely exposure to such situations will be infrequent if at all during your time in practice and risk assessments are carried out in all clinical areas to determine the need for staff and students to complete such training.

However, a more common form of conflict that you will encounter (though just as unreadily) is interpersonal conflict between staff and between staff and service users. Miscommunication and misunderstandings between people will occur; our differing values and opinions, our resistance to change and our dislike for being wrong are all precursors to conflict. Next are six top tips to support your development in this fundamental area of nursing knowledge:

1. *Deal with it*

   Most people tend to avoid conflict. This may seem the simplest and the most gracious thing to do but ignoring it can lead to stress and unresolved feelings of anger or hostility which will impact on your ability to care.

2. *Think it through*

Before addressing the person directly, discuss the situation with an objective third party who can help you clarify the issues, challenge your assumptions and establish how you want to resolve the conflict.

3. *Talk it out, face to face*

Meeting in person is best; it shows respect for the other person and a willingness to resolve the conflict. It also gives each party the opportunity to communicate openly and avoid misunderstandings.

4. *Be prepared to apologise*

Acknowledge your part in creating the conflict and say you are sorry. This is a sign of being a professional, not that you never do anything wrong but you accept responsibility for your behaviour and actions especially when you are in error.

5. *Use a mediator if necessary*

If a situation is particularly difficult and your individual efforts have not worked, you may benefit from the involvement of a mediator. The mediator will remain objective, listen to both sides and facilitate a resolution and compromise.

6. *Work on avoiding conflict*

Take steps to minimise conflict before it happens. Establish good working relationships with colleagues, get to know people and treat everyone with respect. Avoid engaging in gossip or cliques and acknowledge that others may have difficulties that they are struggling to manage which may account for their poor behaviour.

This section has detailed areas of knowledge that are necessary but considered difficult to acquire. The next section will highlight the key psychosocial skill set required for nursing.

Skills

You will hopefully agree that nursing is a highly skilled profession. It is perhaps your main reason for choosing to become a nurse. Being in practice will give you the best opportunity to learn techniques and procedures. However, the skills of a nurse are not just physical skills based on manual dexterity and muscle memory. This section focuses on core nursing skills that should not be neglected at the expense of getting 'hands-on' experience.

Communication

The development of your communication skills will be a necessary component of your nursing practice. While in the CLE you should grasp every opportunity to liaise and communicate with all members of the multidisciplinary team, the service users and their family and friends. In doing so, you will utilise different communication methods and strengthen these skills. Try out Activity 4.5 to identify the different types of communication skills and how well you are developing these in your practice. Be encouraged to seek feedback on your communication style with staff and service users. And use your supernumerary status to spend time just speaking or rather listening to service users. This will help you to develop the following attributes of your communication: being genuine, accepting and empathic (Dahlke et al. 2016). Being in practice will mean you will learn how to adapt your communication with someone who has limited or different communication from you.

Activity 4.5 How well do you communicate?

The different types of communication are:

- **Listening** – that is, really hearing and attending to what someone says.
- **Non-verbal** – that is, your body language (eye contact, facial expression, posture and use of touch) which conveys your level of interest and engagement in the communication that is happening.
- **Verbal** – that is, having clear, accurate and honest spoken communication delivered in an appropriate, kind and respectful manner.
- **Questioning** – that is, using open or closed questions to establish what a service user may want or need.
- **Written** – that is, a written record of the care provided.

For each type of communication answer the following questions:

1. What makes this type of communication easy for you?
2. What makes this type of communication difficult for you?
3. How would you use this form of communication if you were busy?
4. How would you use this form of communication if you were involved in an incident, a complaint or a conflict?
5. How is your demonstration of this type of communication affected when you are observed and when you are on your own?

Record keeping

Aligned with good communication skills is your ability to keep clear and accurate records. Record keeping is covered in Section 10 of The Code (NMC 2015). To achieve this, you must:

10.1 complete all records at the time or as soon as possible after an event, recording if the notes are written some time after the event.

10.2 identify any risks or problems that have arisen and the steps taken to deal with them so that colleagues who use the records have all the information they need.

10.3 complete all records accurately and without any falsification.

10.4 attribute any entries you make in any record to yourself (full name and designation), making sure they are clearly written, dated and timed, and do not include unnecessary abbreviations, jargon or speculation.

10.5 take all steps to make sure that all records are kept securely and confidentially.

Emma's story (Mental Health nursing student)

'I struggled with writing in client notes; it felt like I was either writing too much or not enough. I would read through other people's entries and ask my mentor to check what I had written. Understanding the purpose of record keeping has helped me focus my writing.'

In each placement, you will need to establish the agreed record keeping processes including how to access them and add entries. See Box 4.1 for some top tips on record keeping. Other points to consider include:

➢ How does the record keeping process differ according to the clinical area?

➢ How involved are service users in the development of their records?

➢ Are diaries kept for service users as a record of their stay?

➢ What is the policy on service users accessing their records during an admission and following an admission?

➢ How are records used beyond the immediate care of the service user, for example for purposes of audit, research or investigations?

➢ How are records retrieved during routine hours and out of hours?

➤ How are records produced for a service user who is 'out of area'?

➤ What is the role of information technology in the storage, recording and accessing of records, for example pathology systems, databases, health informatics?

Box 4.1 Five top tips for effective record keeping

1. Avoid subjectivity and remain objective. For example, *'Patient has a temperature of 38.5'* rather than *'The patient feels hot'*.

2. Avoid characterising behaviour or giving an impression. Describe behaviour or write down statements made by the service user or family members. For example, *'Patient smiling, asking staff about their evenings'* rather than *'Appears in good spirits'*.

3. As a rule, use sentences – noun, verb, and adjective and check grammar and spelling. For example, *'Patient coughing productively'* rather than *'Coughing'*; or *'Blood pressure dropped from 110/60 at 0800 to 100/50 at 0815 to 80/40 at 0845'* rather than *'Progressive hypotension'*.

4. Document any recommendations that you make that the service user outright rejects, and document their words. This evidences that you were educating the service user about the need for a treatment, medication, precautions, or to cease an unhealthy habit, but the service user rejected your advice.

5. When documenting an event for an incident report describe the service user's condition, any interventions made, the service user's response to them, and what you observed, if anything. It is best to limit your entries to descriptions of observations and actions, rather than making conclusions about causes.

Care planning

Care planning is the process of identifying the service user's problems and selecting interventions to help resolve or minimise these problems. It enables the care that a nurse provides to be individualised to the needs of the specific service user (Ballantyne 2016). This care may be documented in the form of a care plan or recorded in the notes as an evaluation of the care delivered in the preceding shift. To support the development of your care planning skills use the stages of the nursing process:

➤ Assessment – in this stage you will gather information about the service user's care needs.

➤ Plan – in this stage you will use the information gained from the assessment to plan the care.

➤ Implementation – in this stage you will deliver the care.

➢ Evaluation – in this stage you will evaluate the effectiveness of the plan to meet the service user's care needs.

Activity 4.6 Care planning

Make a list of the service users you have looked after in your last placement; note their conditions and care needs.

How did you identify/assess these?

How did you then manage these care needs?

You may be taught that care planning can be structured around a nursing model. Using a model will ensure that a holistic assessment is carried out in order to identify the psychosocial as well as the physical care needs of the service user. Similarly, it will guide the development of the plan and ensure that all sources of information are incorporated from evidence-based practice, national guidance and local practice, and so on. It will also support the evaluation of the care as it provides a standard of nursing against which the outcome of the care can be measured. See Table 4.4 for examples of nursing models according to nursing field.

Table 4.4   Examples of nursing models according to nursing field

Nursing field	Nursing model
Adult	• Neuman's Systems Model
	• Orem's Self-care Deficit Nursing Theory
	• Roy's Adaptation Model of Nursing
	• Roper–Logan–Tierney's Model for Nursing
Children's	• Mercer's Maternal Role Attainment Theory
	• Kolcaba's Theory of Comfort
	• Casey's Model of Nursing
	• Hilton Davis Family Partnership
Learning Disabilities	• Henderson's Nursing Need Theory
	• Parse's Human Becoming Theory
	• Erickson's Modelling and Role Modelling Theory
	• King's Theory of Goal Attainment
Mental Health	• Barker's Tidal Model of Mental Health Recovery
	• Pender's Health Promotion Model
	• Peplau's Theory of Interpersonal Relations
	• Watson's Philosophy and Science of Caring

Non-technical skills

Non-technical skills are social, cognitive and personal skills that will impact on clinical performance. This term is often associated with the term human factors. Human factors encompass all those factors that can influence people and their behaviour. These include environmental and organisational influences, the nature of the task or procedure and the individual characteristics of the person completing the task (Gordon 2012). Examples of human factors and the associated non-technical skills are listed here.

Human factors

> ➤ workload demands

> ➤ physical/mental demands of the task

> ➤ the design of a device/product

> ➤ the process of the task

> ➤ the physical environment.

Non-technical skills

> ➤ communication

> ➤ teamwork

> ➤ leadership

> ➤ decision making

> ➤ time management

> ➤ situational awareness

> ➤ values and beliefs.

The 'Further reading and resources' section in this chapter has links to recommended websites and videos which will provide you with more detail about integrating human factors into healthcare. As a starting point, complete Activity 4.7.

Activity 4.7 Values clarification exercise (Warfield and Manley 1990)

It is understood that our values and beliefs influence our behaviour. A values clarification exercise can be used to identify our values and beliefs. By making our values

▶

◀

and beliefs explicit we can then develop how to make them a reality in our practice. A match between what we say, what we believe and what we do is one of the hallmarks of effective individuals, teams and organisations.

Spend time completing the following statements.

I believe the ultimate purpose of nursing is ...

I believe this purpose can be achieved by ...

I believe my role in achieving this purpose is ...

I believe the factors that inhibit or enable me to achieve this purpose include ...

Other values and beliefs that I hold about nursing are ...

Management

This is not a skill to be left to learn until you are in year three of the course. The level of autonomy that you will gain as you progress through the course will mean there is a greater expectation that you display management skills in the latter part of the course but management encompasses more than just managing a ward. Consider your day-to-day practice – how do you manage your workload and what factors do you consider help you to prioritise your work? Are you effective at delegating when your workload gets too big? (See the section on 'Knowledge' above, specifically on clinical decision making and delegation.)

This section has focused on the psychosocial rather than the physical care skills you need to learn. If you are concerned about learning the technical skills of a nurse speak with your personal tutor about accessing suitable resources and texts and flag this up with your mentor who will be able to guide your learning in this equally important area. Further topics that would also be helpful for you to explore are end-of-life care, advanced care planning, use of information technology, **sustainability** in healthcare and **safeguarding**. To initiate your learning in these areas refer to the 'Further reading and resources' section at the end of this chapter. Alongside your knowledge and skills the final section of this chapter will detail the attitudes you would need to learn while you are a student.

Attitudes

Having the right attitude is synonymous with the nursing profession. Your attitude will direct your behaviour, your willingness to learn and ensure you demonstrate the required knowledge and skills in a professional manner.

The first consideration in developing the right attitude is to identify with the profession. Being in practice will mean you become 'part' of the profession; it is the start of your socialisation into nursing and the formation of your own nursing identity. It is hoped that you will be surrounded by positive role models, that you will have a sense of belonging to and a confidence in the profession. Socialisation can simply occur through being immersed in the placement – by observing and participating in the activities of the clinical setting. Remember to apply your theory of what nursing is to what you see nurses do. How do their actions match or deviate from your understanding?

Next, take the time to engage in professional dialogue with the wider healthcare team – each member of the team will have undergone a programme of education in order to undertake the role they occupy. What is the role of other professions and how does their work highlight the distinctiveness of nursing? These conversations will also help you to determine how well you identify with being a nurse.

Your professionalism is also bound up in having a person-centred attitude – note, this has superseded the term patient-centred. This means acting deliberately to place the person (who they are, what they want/need, what they don't want/need) at the heart of your nursing practice. The development of this attitude is dependent on purposeful interactions with service users, carers and family. Through these exchanges you will gain a sense of empathy and your role will change from just participating in practice as a learner to engaging in practice as a professional who has the responsibility to puts the interests of service users first, to promote trust through professionalism and to deliver safe and effective care (NMC 2015).

The final aspect is developing an attitude of delivering **ethical practice**. It is important to recognise that even in ordinary and everyday healthcare you will need to make reasoned judgements that consider the ethical elements of a situation. The primary goal in ethical practice is to be competent and then maintain your competence. You will need to be **morally aware** and learn how to act as a moral agent. To support this development you could take key ethical issues as a theme for a day in practice and witness how these are upheld or achieved, and if they are not analyse the reasons why not. Themes could include:

➤ consent

➤ privacy and dignity

➤ decision making

➤ confidentiality

➤ service users as participants in research

➤ withdrawing/withholding treatment

➤ disagreement between a service user/carer/family and the healthcare professional

➤ health inequalities

➤ clinical incident.

The required attitudes of a nurse are linked to developing your professional identity through your socialisation in practice: providing person-centred care by engaging in meaningful interactions with service users, carers and family and displaying ethical practice by adopting moral awareness and competent practice.

Summary

This chapter has focused on what you can learn in practice; it began with a description of the Assessment of Practice document as this will be the primary source of evidencing what you intend to and what you actually learn in practice. Key aspects of the Assessment of Practice document include formation of a learning contract and an action plan.

The three areas of what you need to learn are the required knowledge, skills and attitudes of a nurse. In the first section of the chapter the different types of knowledge were defined and an understanding of nursing theory was given. Specific aspects of knowledge that students struggle to learn were detailed including risk assessment, clinical decision making, delegation and conflict resolution.

The next section explored the psychosocial as opposed to physical skills that you should learn. Some related back to the knowledge section, such as care planning and management, and others were part of the non-technical skills or human factors, such as communication and record keeping. The final section reviewed the attitudes of the nurse and how, through socialisation, focused interactions with service users, carers, family and becoming morally aware, you will develop the appropriate professional identity, person-centred approach and ethical practice.

Knowledge review

See Appendix 4 to compare your answers.

1. What is a learning contract?

2. What is the difference between a learning contact and an action plan?

3. What is a metaparadigm and what are the four specific metaparadigms in nursing?

4. Which section of The Code refers to delegation?

5. Name the human factors and non-technical skills related to healthcare.

6. What term has superseded 'patient-centred' care?

Further reading and resources

Nursing Theory:

McCrae, N. 2012. Whither nursing models? The value of nursing theory in the context of evidence-based practice and multidisciplinary healthcare. *Journal of Advanced Nursing.* 68(1): 222–229.

Nursing Theory – provides examples and full details of nursing models: http://www.nursing-theory.org/theories-and-models/

Evidence-based practice:

National Confidential Enquiry into Patient Outcome and Death (NCEPOD) – the purpose of this organisation is to assist in maintaining and improving standards of care for adults and children by undertaking confidential surveys and research. Areas of research covered by NCEPOD include non-invasive ventilation, young person's mental health and sepsis: http://www.ncepod.org.uk/

Human Factors:

Martin Bromley and Human Factors: https://www.youtube.com/watch?v=JzlvgtPIof4

Clinical Human Factors Group: http://chfg.org/

Patient Safety First – implementing human factors in healthcare: http://www.improvementacademy.org/documents/Projects/human_factors/Human-Factors-How-to-Guide-v1.2.pdf

End of Life Care:

End of Life Care (e-learning package): http://www.e-lfh.org.uk/programmes/end-of-life-care/

End of Life Care NICE quality standard and guidance: https://www.nice.org.uk/guidance/ng31/chapter/Implementation-getting-started

https://www.nice.org.uk/guidance/qs13

National End of Life Care Intelligence Network: http://www.endoflifecare-intelligence.org.uk/home

UK Government End of Life Care policies: https://www.gov.uk/government/policies/end-of-life-care

Advanced Care Planning: http://www.goldstandardsframework.org.uk/advance-care-planning

Dying Matters: http://www.dyingmatters.org/gp_page/
how-help-your-patients-plan

Information Technology:

Information Technology – King's Fund: https://www.kingsfund.org.uk/
time-to-think-differently/trends/information-technologies
UK Government Information Technology: https://www.england.nhs.uk/
digitaltechnology/
https://www.gov.uk/government/news/review-of-information-technolog
y-in-nhs
http://www.ukchip.org/
Digital Literacy: https://www.hee.nhs.uk/our-work/
research-learning-innovation/technology-enhanced-learning/digital-literacy
IT skills (e-learning package): https://www.itskills.nhs.uk/

Sustainability:

NHS Sustainability Plans: https://www.england.nhs.uk/stps/
NHS Sustainable Development Unit: http://www.sduhealth.org.uk/
Sustainability – King's Fund: https://www.kingsfund.org.uk/projects/
environmental-sustainability-health-and-social-care
Centre for Sustainable Healthcare: http://sustainablehealthcare.org.uk/

Safeguarding:

NHS Safeguarding: https://www.england.nhs.uk/ourwork/safeguarding/
Safeguarding – Care Quality Commission: http://www.cqc.org.uk/content/
safeguarding-people
UK Government Safeguarding: https://www.gov.uk/government/publications/
safeguarding-children-and-young-people/safeguarding-children-and-young-
people

5

Who?

Learning outcomes

After reading and completing the activities in this chapter you will be able to:

➤ Identify the different people you can learn from in practice.

➤ Explore the mentor role and their responsibilities to support your learning.

➤ Analyse the benefits and challenges of learning from different people.

➤ Develop strategies to maximise your learning from each person you encounter in practice.

As a student entering the clinical learning environment (CLE) your learning will be supported by a range of different people. This chapter aims to identify who these groups of people are and how to optimise your learning from the time you spend with them. Each group has different reasons to be in practice and this is important to recognise as these reasons may be different to your own. For you, practice is defined as a CLE and your status is supernumerary, that is, your reason to be in practice is to learn.

For the nurse their reason to be in practice is to deliver safe and effective nursing care. This is provided in adherence with The Code (NMC 2015). Within The Code there is an expectation that all nurses will support the learning of students and this is especially so for the nurse who is allocated as your **mentor**. However, the priority in practice for the nurse must always be directed towards the service user(s) rather than your learning. Often, your mentor will skilfully manage this priority while facilitating your learning at the same time. However, you will need to remain attentive to the instances when your needs understandably become of lesser importance in comparison to the clinical demands of the placement. On such occasions, there is still a benefit to you of learning about nursing responsibilities and accountability or using this as an opportunity for independent study.

For the service user their contact with you represents a clinical encounter, whether this occurs in their home, a GP surgery, an outpatient's clinic, a therapy session, a hospital or a hospice and so on. The service user may be acutely unwell physically and/or psychologically, they may even be unconscious and have no recollection of meeting you. Many service users will be very selfless and patient with you. They will often excuse your hesitancy or lack of knowledge and skills. They may even act as the expert to help you understand a specific disease or treatment but more importantly to give you an insight into what this means for them and how the situation in which you meet them is impacting on their life. The principle to remember is that you would not ordinarily have met this person or group of people except in the context of attending the placement. This should be viewed as a privilege to meet strangers, to develop a therapeutic relationship with them and to provide them with nursing care.

For the multidisciplinary team, which will be made up of diverse health and social care professionals, their reasons to be in practice are wide-ranging. Again, the most obvious reason will be linked to direct patient care. However, other reasons for professionals to be in practice will include research, audit, management, leading/team-working, organisational support and clinical governance. These different roles and responsibilities are helpful for you to recognise and appreciate as nurses also work within multidisciplinary teams and it is important to understand the parameters of each professional role and the most effective ways for these teams to work.

In terms of the other nursing students that you will encounter on placement, while you will share a common goal of learning in practice, you are likely to have differing learning needs. This will be increasingly so if, compared to you, your fellow students are in a different nursing field and/or academic year. As a result of being in the same CLE, you may have to negotiate with your peers if you are all trying to access the same learning opportunities, it may be an effort to differentiate yourself from among your peers and you may struggle not to compare yourself and your progress with colleagues who appear to be doing so much better than you. Despite these challenges there are great benefits of learning together with your peers.

As with nursing students it is helpful to consider that other groups of people may also be in practice to learn. A registered nurse, for example, may be learning a new skill, a service user may be receiving health education and students from other healthcare professions may also be present in the CLE.

Hannah's story (Children's nursing student)

'I was so enthusiastic to go out into practice. I had a list of things I wanted to see and to learn about. But once I got into practice I realised not everyone else was interested in my learning. I had to mould my learning to what was happening at the time. I had a great mentor who wanted to help me get through my list but I realised that it was not going to be possible and that I needed to understand more about what I could learn from the people in practice as this was real-time nursing which was much better than my list of what nurses do and therefore what I thought I should learn.'

In this chapter, we will explore the benefits and challenges to your learning of meeting different groups of people in the CLE, namely nurses, service users, members of the multidisciplinary team and your fellow students.

The nurse

The **Nursing and Midwifery Council** (NMC) has established four developmental stages for nurses to support and assess learning in practice. These are set out in the document *Standards to Support Learning and Assessment in Practice* (NMC 2008).

Stage 1 applies to all nurses. *The Code: Professional Standards and Behaviour for Nurses and Midwives* (NMC 2015) requires every nurse to adhere to the following:

➤ support students' and colleagues' learning to help them develop their professional competence and confidence (Section 9.4). [...]
➤ act as a role model of professional behaviour for students and newly registered nurses and midwives to aspire (Section 20.8).

Stage 2 applies to nurses who become mentors. A mentor will have successfully completed an NMC-approved mentor programme in order to support and assess you in practice and confirm that you are capable of safe and effective practice. A sign-off mentor must make the final assessment of your practice to confirm that you have met the required competencies for entry to the NMC professional nursing register.

Stage 3 applies to nurses who become practice teachers. A practice teacher will normally already be a mentor and will have successfully completed an NMC-approved practice teacher programme in order to support and assess students undertaking a programme leading to registration as a specialist community public health nurse (SCPHN).

Stage 4 applies to nurses who become teachers. A teacher will be based in higher education and will have successfully completed an NMC-approved teacher programme in order to support and assess students undertaking a programme leading to registration as a nurse or a post-registration qualification.

As a student in the CLE you are there to learn to become a nurse and therefore you should be mainly working with and learning from nurses. Nursing roles are highly varied and thus the knowledge and skills you will learn from nurses in different roles will enhance your practice, develop your appreciation of the complexity of nursing and encourage you in your future career path. Table 5.1 presents examples of the different nursing job titles you may come across while on placement. Which were you already familiar with? How could you access nurses in roles you have less knowledge or awareness of?

While all nurses should be willing to support your learning and assess your practice, the NMC specifically requires all students on an NMC-approved pre-registration nursing education programme to be allocated to a mentor. See Box 5.1 for key information on the mentor's role. In addition to being allocated a mentor you may also have a buddy or associate mentor who will be a registered nurse undertaking their mentor qualification. A team approach to mentoring will often result in a better learning experience for you as there are more people available to facilitate your learning. It can also avoid the issue of subjectivity in assessment as the decision to confirm if you are competent is based on the comprehensive

Table 5.1 Nursing job titles according to domains

	Primary/Community	Acute	Specialist
Clinical	practice nurse community nurse health visitor	staff nurse clinical nurse specialist advanced nurse nurse consultant	occupational health nurse prison nurse school nurse
Leader	community (deputy) sister/charge nurse community matron	(deputy) sister/charge nurse matron	(deputy) head nurse chief nursing officer
Educator	link nurse practice teacher education lead	link nurse practice education facilitator education lead	lecturer-practitioner senior lecturer principal lecturer
Researcher	clinical trials nurse clinical research nurse reader professor		

supervision of a number of nurses rather than just one individual – note, your mentor will talk with their nursing colleagues about you to determine the level of your knowledge, skills and attitude.

Box 5.1 The role of the mentor

- While giving direct care at least 40% of a student's time must be spent being supervised (directly or indirectly) by a mentor.

- When on a final placement this 40% of the student's time is in addition to the protected time (one hour per week) to be spent with a sign-off mentor.

- Mentors should not normally support more than three students at any one time.

- An ongoing achievement record including comments from mentors must be passed from one placement to the next to enable judgements to be made on the student's progress.

- In the final placement of a pre-registration programme, mentors are required either to be a sign-off mentor or supported by a sign-off mentor or a practice teacher in order to make final decisions on competency.

The role of the mentor is divided in to eight domains. Each domain is identified in this section in order to help you understand the mentor's role and how they will work with you to support your learning in practice.

Establishing effective working relationships

From the student's perspective an effective working relationship with the mentor is undoubtedly the most important aspect of the mentor's role (Esmaeili et al. 2014). The behaviour of the mentor towards you as a student let alone a service user will shape your idea of the kind of nurse you want to become (see Activity 5.1).

Activity 5.1 Are you impressed or depressed?

If you have worked with one or more mentor(s) think about who impressed you. What was it about them that made you want to emulate them?

What about the mentor(s) who depressed you? What was it about them that made you not want to emulate them?

See Chapter 3 for strategies on how to manage difficult relationships with your mentor.

If your mentor is welcoming, friendly and builds your confidence your learning is much more effective. Conversely, if your mentor is discouraging or limits your participation in activities this will have a detrimental effect on your learning and progress. Refer to the section 'The prerequisites of the CLE' in Chapter 2 – 'Where?' – and to the section 'You have the ability to learn' in Chapter 3 – 'How?' – for details on managing issues with your mentor and the support available to you. The characteristics of a good mentor are those which enable or promote your learning as compared to disabling characteristics which will restrict your learning and impede your motivation to learn.

➤ *Enabling characteristics of a mentor include being*: professional, organised, caring, self-confident, present and involved should anything untoward arise for the student, a positive role model, a good communicator.

➤ *Disabling characteristics of a mentor include being*: a negative role model, role conflict, poor practice, lack of availability due to time constraints, workload pressures or attitude, a poor communicator.

The communication between you and your mentor is vital for an effective working relationship. You will need to make sure that what your mentor communicates to you is clear and that you clarify the meaning if you are unsure. This may also require you to be confident to say no or to question the mentor if you are uncertain about what to do or say in a given situation. Try out Activity 5.2 to determine your own list of positive characteristics for a mentor.

Activity 5.2 Positive characteristics of a mentor?

When you are in practice and working with a range of mentors, make a note of the qualities you feel make a good nurse and mentor. Consider how you could integrate these qualities into your own practice.

Frank's story (Adult nursing student)

'Sometimes I was really pleased to be able to start afresh without people having pre-conceived ideas about me. Other times I found it a bit tedious. The mentors who took the time to get to know me and read previous comments in the practice book were much better. The best mentors really wanted to know why I wanted to become a nurse.'

The mentor will also be integral in helping you form effective relationships with others. Your mentor is likely to be a member of a team and the greater your integration in to the team, the better your sense of belonging – feeling valued, trusted and respected. Again, this will have a positive influence on your learning. Invariably you will be allocated to a different practice area with each placement. Therefore, every time you enter a new CLE you will have to start afresh forming relationships with a new team. Each team will have differing compositions and goals and these variations can make feeling part of the team that bit more difficult to establish. Box 5.2 has information to help facilitate your assimilation into a team.

Box 5.2 How to fit into a team?

Here are some suggestions on how to better negotiate your integration into a team:

Be familiar with the structure and purpose of the team
It can be helpful to identify if there is a hierarchy in the team. What roles are represented in the team? More specifically, how are nurses represented in the team? Observe the interactions and dynamics of the team to help you understand how the team functions. What are the goals of the team?

Be authentic in your interactions with team members
It is understandable to feel nervous when joining a new group and this can mean we behave as we think others would want. However, this is not a good approach to take when forming honest working relationships. Just make sure to respect people's boundaries, and always behave professionally.

Be realistic about being a team member
As you are a student, you may not have lots of experience and you will not be staying in the team for long. But these should not be barriers or reasons to exclude you from the team. The team should understand the transitory nature of your involvement in the team and still be able to accommodate this.

Be supportive of the team
It is important to avoid criticising the team or how the team works. You may not know why certain things are done in a particular way. Consider how you can assimilate established processes and participate in team activities.

Facilitation of learning

A mentor is required to facilitate your time in the CLE. Therefore, you need to make sure that you are clear with your mentor about what stage you are at on the course. What have you already learnt? What are you currently learning? What are you struggling to learn? This will help them select appropriate learning opportunities to meet your learning needs.

In addition, it is likely that your mentor will utilise a range of teaching and learning strategies to facilitate your learning. As a result you should be prepared to try out ways of learning that may be less familiar to you. The choice of strategy will be dependent on the area of practice you are in, your agreed learning needs and your level of experience or competence. Chapter 3 – 'How?' – provides more details on learning strategies.

One of the great benefits of working with your mentor is that your learning will often be one-to-one. The teaching at university will be delivered in a range of formats – you may attend large group teaching in a lecture theatre with the rest of your cohort, which could potentially comprise a couple of hundred students. Other sessions may be in smaller groups, particularly if a skill is being taught and the opportunity to practise is available. Very rarely in the academic setting will you be fortunate enough to receive one-to-one teaching, but this is something that you will benefit from in clinical practice.

One-to-one teaching may take place in a number of settings within the clinical area. It can be argued that the best teaching occurs at the 'bedside' where either you observe or participate in the delivery of direct care. Depending upon the stage of education you are at, your mentor will encourage you to take the lead under their direct or indirect supervision.

Assessment and accountability

A significant part of the mentor's role is their assessment of your competence. Your mentor is accountable for confirming that you have or have not met the NMC competencies in practice. If you are a final-year student on your final placement you will be assigned a sign-off mentor who will be required to confirm that you have or have not met the NMC standards of competence for entry to the register and that you are capable of safe and effective practice. Integral to being assessed is receiving feedback. If you are not doing well in the placement, the mentor will manage this so that you can understand why you are failing and help you to enhance your practice in future placements. Your assessments and feedback should be captured in your Assessment of Practice document. See Chapter 4 – 'What?' – for more details on the document and Chapter 6 – 'When?' – for a detailed section on assessment as a means of learning.

Your mentor is also accountable for planning and coordinating your learning experience and determining the amount of either direct or indirect supervision that you will require. Your mentor will use their professional judgement and local/national policy to determine which activities they consider safe to delegate to you as a student. It is important to remember that your mentor is accountable for their decisions and for ensuring public safety and trust. Therefore, you will need to respect their decisions and accept any request from the mentor that they observe your practice first before allowing you to undertake the same task or activity independently. See Table 5.2 which outlines the differences between direct and indirect supervision and the related teaching and learning activities.

Table 5.2 Direct and indirect supervision by mentor

Direct supervision by mentor	
Learning strategy	**Rationale**
Role modelling Student to observe in practice as directed by the nurse in performance of skill and/or role	1. The student can be orientated to the CLE 2. The student can encounter the reality of practice in a non-threatening way 3. The student can receive technical explanations and rationales
Coaching Student to assist in practice as directed by the nurse in performance of skill and/or role	1. The student can focus on key aspects of practice to according to their learning needs 2. The student can be supported in complex tasks 3. The student can be alerted to areas of practice where mistakes could easily be made
Participation Student to participate in practice as directed by the nurse in performance of skill and/or role	1. The student can gain confidence in their own practice 2. The student can identify areas of their practice that require improvement or development
Indirect supervision by mentor	
Learning strategy	**Rationale**
Facilitated discussion Student to participate in facilitated discussion with mentor prior to performance of skill and/or role	1. The student can prepare for what is expected of them 2. The student can review their risk assessment strategy 3. The student can explore their knowledge and skill in a range of potential scenarios
Participation Student to participate in practice in performance of skill and/or role	1. The student can select activities within their capability but also be challenged to develop their competence in new areas 2. The student can determine their level of competence 3. The student can develop autonomous practice
Reflection Student to reflect on/in practice in performance of skill and/or role	1. The student can think through their practice to gain further understanding/meaning 2. The student can develop critical thinking skills

Evaluation of learning

Your mentor should be responsive to making changes to your learning arising from the evaluation of your experiences in practice. Evaluation can occur at any time during or more commonly after the placement although there are limited direct benefits to you if you only evaluate the placement once you have left. Box 5.3 is an example of an evaluation form to be completed at the end of the placement period. However, the statements can be used equally to prompt you to evaluate during your placement as well. For example, if reflecting on your experience in practice you note that you have not received any feedback on your practice, you could address this formally in a midway meeting or informally during ongoing interactions with your mentor. Changes in how your mentor works and supports your learning can be difficult to accomplish if:

➢ you are not engaged in monitoring progress in your own learning

➢ you find it hard to communicate your learning needs

➢ you have no opportunity to or confidence in offering feedback to your mentor.

Box 5.3 Placement evaluation (example)

Preparation and Orientation	Response	
I accessed information about the placement prior to starting	Yes	No
I contacted the placement prior to starting	Yes	No
My arrival was expected	Yes	No
I was orientated to the placement within the first three days	Yes	No
I was told my mentor's name before or on the first day	Yes	No
I met with my mentor in the first week to plan my learning	Yes	No
Comments/reflections:		
Assessment and Development	Response	
My mentor gave me regular constructive feedback	Yes	No
I met with my mentor at the midway to review my learning	Yes	No

▶

◄

I met with my mentor at the end to review my progress	Yes	No
My mentor understood the assessment document	Yes	No
I understood the assessment document	Yes	No
The assessments were achievable in this placement	Yes	No
I was able to access information services within the Trust	Yes	No
I discussed with my mentor any issues/problems	Yes	No

Comments/reflections:

Clinical Learning Environment	**Response**	
I was able to discuss learning opportunities with my mentor	Yes	No
I was encouraged to participate in service user care	Yes	No
I was able to participate in interprofessional working	Yes	No
The evidence base of the care delivered was explained	Yes	No
I had staff support in accessing learning resources	Yes	No
I felt valued while on the placement	Yes	No
The placement area was conducive to learning	Yes	No

Comments/reflections:

Overall comments

Positive aspects of the placement:

Areas of the placement that could be improved:

Enter up to five words that summarise your experience of this placement:

1.

2.

3.

4.

5.

Creating an environment for learning

As outlined in Chapter 2 – 'Where?' – each placement that you enter becomes for you a CLE, whereas for your mentor it is first and foremost their place of work. Therefore, your mentor must negotiate their teaching and assessing role alongside their nursing role. Your mentor will most likely have established set learning outcomes that can be achieved within the specific CLE. These should not be to the exclusion of your own personal goals and learning needs but rather this approach should reassure you that you mentor views their workplace as a CLE and has designed learning activities for you in advance.

While working with your mentor in the CLE ensure you focus as much on learning problem solving, critical thinking and clinical decision making skills as the practical tasks. Consider how well your mentor tests your ability to problem-solve or to make decisions using your prior knowledge, the available assessment findings and local/national policy and guidance. This approach to learning will enable you to develop your autonomy and accountability.

James' story (Mental health nursing student)

'I pestered my mentors all the time to challenge and question me. I did not want to waste time on placement just learning skills that I could pick up after I was registered. I wanted to use the safety net of being supervised and supernumerary to test out what nursing is all about. How to communicate with different people: professionals and patients? How to really make a difference in a patient's life and figure out how to do this with lots of patients with competing demands?'

Context of practice

The emphasis on this element of the role is the mentor's contribution to ensuring safe and effective practice is fostered, implemented, evaluated and disseminated in the CLE. It may come as a surprise but your mentor will not be 'the all-knowing expert'. While they will hopefully be able to impart their knowledge and skills readily there may be occasions when they need to undertake their own learning and research to support either your learning or their own professional development. This is a great opportunity for you to observe how registered nurses develop their knowledge and skills further. Is it through personal study, liaison with colleagues, attendance at study days or a combination of these learning approaches? How does your mentor initiate and respond to practice developments? How are they made aware of the latest practices? How does your mentor learn?

Evidence-based practice

Following on from the context of practice it is imperative that your mentor is able to apply research to and identify an evidence-base for their nursing practice. Having knowledge, experience and an interest in the nursing profession are seen by many students as the most important factors. Having up-to-date knowledge and being able to answer student questions are key characteristics of effective mentorship.

Leadership

Leadership is an important quality for a mentor even if they are a band 5 and have no managerial responsibility. Within this role the mentor is responsible for planning learning experiences that meet your defined learning needs. Your mentor will act as an advocate to support you in accessing learning opportunities. They will need to prioritise their work to accommodate the support of students within their role and feedback on the effectiveness of learning and assessment in practice.

While being a mentor will benefit their own personal well-being and professional development it is important to acknowledge the work and effort that a mentor puts in to support your learning. Thanking your mentor and letting them know how their mentoring has helped you in your understanding of how to become a nurse are great examples of positive feedback. Perhaps your course has a 'Mentor of the Year' nomination or other ways to acknowledge excellent mentors. Consider who you could put forward. Even if they are not successful just knowing that they have been nominated can be a great boost and motivation to continue mentoring. Remember, one day, you too are likely to become a mentor and will appreciate the thanks from your students.

The service user

The term 'service user' refers to the patient or client, that is, the person that receives your nursing care. Both within the theory and practice of nursing the person is at the centre of this care giving (Lee and Fawcett 2013). The service user and how they are nursed, which according to the

NMC is safely and effectively, should be the focus and motivation for your learning. By recognising the unique contribution of the service user to your learning you will be better able to develop your professional nursing role.

Most healthcare settings are linked to educational institutions, for example, University Hospital NHS Trusts and these organisations will have charters or statements which establish the healthcare setting as a place where service users are to expect their care to be part of a learning experience for a healthcare student both at pre-registration and post-registration level. Similarly, your university may have a public and service user forum which will guide and monitor service user involvement in your nursing education. You may want to identify if these provisions exist in your practice areas and university.

The rationale for service user involvement in your learning

The recommendation for service user involvement in student learning has been acknowledged by all healthcare-related **professional, statutory and regulatory bodies** (PSRBs). Specifically within nursing education the NMC requires programme providers to evidence how service users and carers contribute to the development of the **curriculum**, the learning experience and the assessment of nursing students.

The service user may come from a very different background to you and therefore you need to be able to practise competently within a multi-ethnic, diverse society. **Cultural sensitivity** refers to the ability to care for people from a range of cultural backgrounds. This may include addressing racism or the effects of healthcare discrimination. Worryingly, the health inequalities experienced by minority ethnic groups in the UK are attributed in part to social exclusion and racism within healthcare (Merrell and Olumide 2014). Try out Activity 5.3 to familiarise yourself with what The Code (NMC 2015) says about your role in advocating for service users and challenging inequalities.

Activity 5.3

Read through *The Code: Professional Standards of Practice and Behaviour for Nurses and Midwives* (NMC 2015). Which sections relate to advocating for service users and challenging health inequalities?

How will this inform your learning in practice?

Section 3 of The Code requires the nurse to make sure that people's physical, social and psychological needs are assessed and responded to. Subsection 3.3 necessitates that the nurse acts in partnership with those receiving care, helping them to access relevant health and social care, information and support when they need it. Subsection 3.4 states that the nurse must act as an advocate for the vulnerable, challenging poor practice and discriminatory attitudes and behaviour relating to their care.

Section 1 of The Code requires a nurse to treat people as individuals and uphold their dignity. Specifically subsection 1.5 states that the nurse must respect and uphold people's **human rights**. Box 5.4 details the human rights protected by UK law in the **Human Rights Act 1998**.

Box 5.4 Human rights as protected by UK law

- The right to life

- The prohibition of torture and inhuman treatment

- Protection against slavery and forced labour

- The right to liberty and freedom

- The right to a fair trial and no punishment without law

- Respect for privacy and family life and the right to marry

- Freedom of thought, religion and belief

- Free speech and peaceful protest

- No discrimination regardless of gender, race, sexuality, religion or age

---

When reviewing these rights a number have a more overt link to healthcare provision. During your time in practice you will encounter the difficulties in upholding these rights for individual service users or be confronted with situations when these right(s) are not protected. This is a key learning opportunity for you to understand the rights that every human has particularly while they are in one of the most vulnerable positions as a service user.

The right to life – this means that nobody can try to end a person's life.

Challenges in practice related to this right have focused on assisted dying and the withdrawing and withholding of treatment. At present, in the UK, it is still illegal for anyone to assist in the deliberate act of or to encourage another person to kill themselves. Therefore the right to life does not include the right to die.

Pretty v United Kingdom [2002]

'A woman suffering from an incurable degenerative disease wanted to control when and how she died. To avoid an undignified death, she wanted her husband to help her take her life. She sought assurance that he would not be prosecuted, but the European Court of Human Rights ruled against her challenge.'

Prohibition of inhuman treatment – this means no serious physical or psychological abuse should occur in a health or care setting.

Challenges in practice related to this right include issues of institutional abuse and the quality assurance of the care provided. It also includes reporting concerns in practice about the care provided.

Respect for privacy – this means you have the right to determine who sees you/your body and who knows about you/your body.

Challenges in practice related to this right include maintaining privacy and dignity and gaining consent from service users. Remember that a service user is under no obligation to accept your care. This can be difficult to accept if the only reason they refuse is because you are a student. Maintaining confidentiality, personal information about service users (including official records, photographs, letters, diaries and medical records) should be kept securely and not shared except in certain circumstances.

No discrimination regardless of the person's characteristics or beliefs – this means that a person is not treated less favourably than another person in a similar situation or the person is not disadvantaged by being treated the same as another person when their circumstances are different (for example, if the person is disabled or pregnant).

Challenges in practice related to this right include individualising the care of each patient regardless of, for example, their age, their illness or their ability to communicate. This can be a challenge when you are caring for people too young to be able to communicate or who have difficulties in communicating, for example if they have dementia or even just speak a different language to you.

It is important to understand that the Human Rights Act (1998) does not protect from discrimination in all areas of life – there are other laws that offer more general protection, such as the Equality Act 2010. The Equality Act (2010) subsumed and supersedes previously related legislation such as the Race Relations Act 1976 and the Disability Discrimination Act 1995. The act ensures that health and care organisations must not discriminate against people who have particular protected characteristics.

Protected characteristics

➢ age

➢ disability

➢ gender reassignment

➢ pregnancy and maternity (which includes breastfeeding)

➢ race

➢ religion or belief

➢ sex

➢ sexual orientation

Discrimination

Discrimination, that is, treating some people worse than others because of a protected characteristic, can take a number of different forms:

Direct discrimination – a nurse must not treat a person worse than someone else because of one or more protected characteristics or because they are associated with a person who has a protected characteristic.

> **For example:** A small privately run homecare provider refuses to assist an older client at home because they discover that the older person's partner is HIV positive. This is almost certainly direct discrimination because of disability based on the client's association with a disabled person.

Indirect discrimination – a nurse must not do something to a person who has a particular protected characteristic which would have a worse impact on them than on people who do not share that characteristic.

For example: A disabled person who is a wheelchair user has a hospital appointment but is refused a consultation in a small consultation room as the wheelchair takes up a lot of room. They are interviewed in a curtained cubicle near the public waiting area, but this provides much less privacy than a consultation room. The person is treated unfavourably because of their use of the wheelchair, which is something arising from their disability.

➤ **Victimisation** – a nurse must not treat a person badly because they have complained about discrimination or helped someone else complain.

For example: A patient supports another person's complaint that a GP's surgery has unlawfully discriminated against them. The patient is later told that they will have to find a new GP.

➤ **Harassment** – a nurse must not harass a person.

For example: A member of a service provider's support staff is verbally abusive to a service user in relation to a protected characteristic.

Upholding each person's human rights, avoiding discrimination and maintaining equality in the care delivered is often most challenging when the person you are nursing is unable to make their own decisions. Box 5.5 has a list of reasons why someone may lack capacity. The list does not reflect all groups of service users nor does it conclude that everyone with a mental health disorder or a learning disability would automatically lack capacity.

Box 5.5 Reasons a person *may* lack capacity

If they have:

- a stroke or brain injury
- a mental health disorder
- dementia
- a learning disability
- confusion, drowsiness or are unconsciousness because of an illness or the treatment for it
- substance misuse

The legislation that supports the care of people who lack capacity to make all or some decisions for themselves is the Mental Capacity Act (2005). This act applies to everyone aged over 16, to each decision needing to be made individually and is underpinned by five principles. Principles 1–3 will support the process before or at the point of determining whether someone lacks capacity (Box 5.6 details the two-stage test to determine capacity). Once you have decided that capacity is lacking, principles 4 and 5 are used to support the decision making process.

Box 5.6 Assessing capacity two-stage test

The Mental Capacity Act (2005) contains a two-stage test of capacity:

- Is there an impairment of, or disturbance to, the functioning of the mind or brain?

And if so:

- Is the impairment or disturbance sufficient that the person is unable to make that particular decision?

The act says that a person is unable to make a decision if unable to:

- understand the information relevant to the decision
- retain the information
- use or weigh the information
- communicate his or her decision (by any means)

Principle 1: A presumption of capacity

Every adult has the right to make his or her own decisions and must be assumed to have capacity to do so unless it is proved otherwise. This means that you cannot assume that someone cannot make a decision for themselves just because they have a particular medical condition or disability.

Principle 2: Individuals being supported to make their own decisions

A person must be given all practicable help before anyone treats them as not being able to make their own decisions. This means you should make every effort to encourage and support people to make the decision for themselves. If lack of capacity is established, it is still important that you involve the person as far as possible in making decisions.

Principle 3: Unwise decisions

People have the right to make decisions that others might regard as unwise or eccentric. You cannot treat someone as lacking capacity for this reason. Everyone has their own values, beliefs and preferences which may not be the same as those of other people.

Principle 4: Best interests

Anything done for or on behalf of a person who lacks mental capacity must be done in their best interests.

Principle 5: Less restrictive option

Someone making a decision or acting on behalf of a person who lacks capacity must consider whether it is possible to decide or act in a way that would interfere less with the person's rights and freedoms of action, or whether there is a need to decide or act at all. Any intervention should be weighed up in the particular circumstances of the case.

Children and young people under 16 years are not included in the above legislation. It is the person who has 'parental responsibility' who will consent on behalf of the child, such as the child's mother or father, the child's legally adopted guardian or a local authority designated to care for the child. However, a young person under 16 may have capacity to make decisions, depending on their maturity and ability to understand what is involved. See the 'Further reading and resources' section for information on establishing consent according to the Gillick competency test.

The practice of service user involvement in your learning

The practice of service user involvement in your learning has two key elements. The first is ensuring you are safe in your practice when delivering care to service users and the second is acknowledging the individual in every care activity – currently, there is a move towards person-centred care rather than patient-centred care. This reinforces the idea that the patient is not the sum total of the person and that it is important to maintain a human relationship with the person rather than the management of a collection of signs and symptoms.

As a student it can be problematic to combine person-centred care with the rigours of **patient safety** (Tonks et al. 2014). To maintain compassion and dignity in your care when you are learning new knowledge and skills can be difficult. This struggle is often reinforced by the approach taken on your course particularly in the first year. Your course most likely started with a greater focus on patient safety than person-centred care, for example you will have needed to complete occupational health, disclosure and barring service (DBS) clearance, mandatory training and clinical skills such as hand hygiene and physical measurements before you are even allowed into practice. Similarly, when you are in practice you will be expected to ask for help and to only undertake tasks when you are observed and/or competent to do so. This approach is designed to safeguard you and the service user and to help you settle in and learn in a supportive environment.

However, this can also limit your performance and progress and make it difficult for you to reconcile the notion of person-centred care with the risk of causing harm or deviating from standardised care pathways and the necessary completion of documentation to evidence this. As a result the individual patient and their needs – the premise of person-centred care – start to jar with the objective of standardised approaches to practice. A simple example can be seen in the meeting of personal hygiene needs where the patient wishes to shower in privacy and his falls risk assessment suggests otherwise. By acknowledging this dilemma in your practice and discussing solutions with your mentor and even better the service user themselves you will develop a more comprehensive understanding of nursing and its complexity.

The benefits of service user involvement in your learning

By participating in the care of service users through observation or direct contact it validates your student role and your learning. Interestingly, a study by Barksby (2014) confirmed that service users were largely positive about student nurses and the care they received from them. There is an authenticity to what you will experience as a student in your interactions with and care of service users which cannot be replicated in the classroom setting or simulation suite. You will get to know yourself better, the level of your knowledge, skills and attitudes, your professionalism, your resilience and your ability to respond appropriately to patients who are in pain, confused, anxious and so on.

You will learn how to personalise the care that you provide ('every time for every service user') by having an interest in the person, finding out their unique perspective and needs. You will develop empathy and your ability to communicate to make you better able to negotiate and provide better care. The care of a person will also challenge your assumptions and stereotypes enabling you to develop a non-judgemental and open approach to caring for people.

By being with real people and dealing with real situations, the learning that results is often the most memorable and impactful. At times this learning can be difficult when you encounter people and their circumstances/experiences that are troubling or complex. You will need to develop strategies to deal with situations that distress or challenge your values and beliefs, your knowledge and skills. Activities 5.4 and 5.5 are designed to help you reflect on your encounters with service users and to consider the learning you have gained.

Activity 5.4 Reflecting on feedback from a service user

It is likely that during your time in practice you will receive much unsolicited feedback from service users about the standard of your practice and care. This can be supplemented by more formal engagement in a process of reflection on service user feedback. Most students are able to identify a change in behaviour they have adopted as a result of feedback.

- Plan to carry out a care activity with a service user.

- Ask your mentor to request feedback from the service user on your care (this is a safeguarding measure to avoid putting you and/or the service user in a vulnerable position).

- Your mentor will gain feedback from the service user and relay this back to you.

- Reflect on what you have heard – Is it positive? What you expected? Is it hard to hear or surprising?

- Capture this reflection and work on how you will respond to this. How will your practice be maintained or develop further?

Activity 5.5 Your experience of service user and carer involvement in your learning

Reflect on your experiences of service user and carer involvement in your learning and answer the following questions:

- How does input from service users and carers differ for you from other teaching and learning experiences?

- How have you used these experiences to build your knowledge and practice of nursing?

- How have these experiences helped you gain knowledge and practice that you could not have got in any other way?

- How have these experiences affected the way you approach service users and carers?

The multidisciplinary team

Within the CLE you will work alongside not just your mentor or other nurses but also a range of health and social care professionals – the multi-disciplinary/multiprofessional team. See Activity 5.6 to help you identify members of this team other than nurses, nurse matrons, nurse consultants, nurse specialists and so on.

Activity 5.6 Multidisciplinary team membership

List the members of the multidisciplinary team that you have met or expect to meet.

Healthcare professional	Social care/other professional
e.g. Doctor	e.g. Social worker

From the above list, what kind of working relationship will you have with this professional?

Have you had clinical conversations about patient care with any of the above professionals?

If yes, what was this experience like?

If not, how can you prepare and arrange for this to happen?

Learning from the multidisciplinary team is related to a specific teaching theory called interprofessional learning (IPL).

Definition of interprofessional learning (IPL)

The Centre for the Advancement of Interprofessional Education (CAIPE) has defined IPL as professionals learning with, from and about each other to improve collaboration and quality of care. The ideal is to have multi-disciplinary practice development teams – have you encountered this in your practice area?

The strengths of IPL are in the sharing of teaching and learning resources, fostering a culture of awareness and respect for each profession, improving communication between professions and professionals and

Table 5.3 Examples of interprofessional learning (IPL) activities

Activity	Example	Rationale
Observation and reflection of other professions' clinical practice	• Shadow a foundation doctor during their on-call period • Attend surgery (theatres, endoscopy, maternity) • Attend a clinic (outpatients, GP) • Attend a therapy session	This will provide you with an insight into the demands of the professional's work
Observation and reflection of liaison and communication between professions	• Attend a ward round • Attend a multidisciplinary team meeting • Attend a case conference/ Morbidity and Mortality meeting	This will provide you with an understanding of the shared language and goals of the team and the importance of clear communication between different professions
Participation in and reflection on clinical practice	• Provide care to a service user with another professional • Develop a care plan with one or more other professions	This will provide you with an opportunity for collaborative teamwork and an appreciation of the different roles
Work with administrative and service provision staff	• Arrange a patient transfer • Order medical loan equipment • Request medical records	This will provide you with skills of organisation, delegation and an ability to manage your workload and prioritise care when you require additional staff to support the delivery of care

addressing stereotyping. A final strength is an increased appreciation of each other's priorities and demands in the care of the patient. Table 5.3 provides examples of IPL activities.

The limitations of IPL are that other disciplines may not have the same knowledge base as you and therefore may be less able to support you in your learning about your own profession.

Process of interprofessional learning (IPL)

There are two broad methods of achieving IPL:

➢ Common learning – a range of professionals learn about the same subject, for example diabetes.

➢ Comparative learning – each professional learns about one another's professional involvement in the care of a patient, for example care of a person with diabetes.

Create opportunities to engage in communication with other disciplines. This could be through clinical events, such as a ward round, or informal teaching. For example, a junior doctor may be willing to talk you through a procedure or test result. You could attend a case conference or multidisciplinary team (MDT) meeting which will help you see how the provision of health and social care is structured and the common goal that all professionals have of providing care and services that are in the best interest of each service user.

Using the service user pathway as a model you can plan out your IPL (see Figures 5.1, 5.2, 5.3 and 5.4). First identify the different multidisciplinary team roles that you will encounter in your placement. Secondly, by considering the professionals that are involved before and after the service user enters the placement organise **spoke experiences** (see Chapter 2) to broaden your understanding of the multiplicity of professions that the service user may interact with.

It is important to identify learning outcomes for your IPL. This will give you a specific focus for your learning and ensure that your time with another professional is purposive. Examples of IPL learning outcomes include:

➤ Understand the roles and responsibilities of another professional.

➤ Understand the similarities and differences between professions.

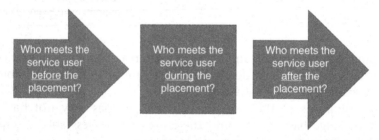

Figure 5.1   Service user pathway (template)

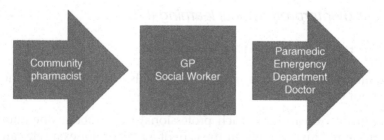

Figure 5.2   Community care example

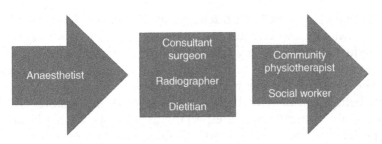

Figure 5.3 Acute care example

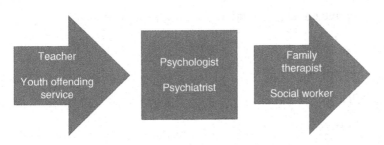

Figure 5.4 Mental health example (Child and Adolescent Mental Health Services)

➤ Understand stereotyping and professional prejudices and the impact of these on interprofessional working.

➤ Demonstrate a set of knowledge, skills, competencies and attitudes that are common to all professions and that underpin the delivery of care.

➤ Develop teamwork skills and improved knowledge of the nature of multidisciplinary teamwork.

➤ Respect, understand and support the roles of other professionals.

➤ Make an effective contribution as an equal member of an interprofessional team.

➤ Collaborate with other professionals in practice.

The student

Learning among students is also known as peer learning and is based on the idea that students learn with, and from, each other without the immediate intervention of the mentor. Students who participate in peer learning have increased confidence and abilities in cooperation and teamwork. It can also counter the complaint that many students report of being just an onlooker. By taking the initiative and caring for patients together students assume responsibility and develop their professional role. The presence of the mentor provides students with the advantage of being confident in their supervised work but enables the mentor to remain clinically active especially as mentors are rarely provided with protected time to spend with students. Being required to provide knowledge and skills means that students take seriously the importance of research and ensuring they have up-to-date information to base their care on.

The positive effects for students are an increase in:

➤ cognitive skills

➤ self-confidence

➤ self-efficacy

➤ autonomy

➤ clinical reasoning/critical thinking

➤ clinical skills

➤ self-evaluation skills

➤ collaborative working

➤ leadership skills

(Carey et al. 2016)

Students are also supported in their learning because they work and learn together. Students undergoing similar experiences are able to support one another and this approach markedly decreases students' reported levels of anxiety. The possibility of asking a peer rather than a mentor if you do not know something also alleviates concerns about being thought of as an awkward student.

Difficulties in student learning arise when students do not want to complete clinical tasks together, or they are unhappy about having to share the mentor's time and attention or having less time to practice independently. These can be easily managed within the placement and it often works best with students in different academic years or even fields. Activity 5.7 offers some examples of peer learning exercises that can be completed while you are in practice.

Activity 5.7 Peer learning exercises

1. If you are on a placement with one or more other nursing students or there are nursing students located in practice settings close by ask a small group to observe your mentor or another clinician completing a care activity.

   Following the activity as a group deconstruct what you observed. What did each of you focus on? Was it the same or different?

   It can also be helpful to critique the practice – can you agree as a group what was effective and why? What could be improved and why?

2. Share the care of a service user with another nursing student – How do you delegate? How do you communicate? How is the service user involved in their care? Are you both at the same level of knowledge, skill and attitude?

3. Ask your mentor to set you and your colleague(s) a challenge that you will need to work collaboratively together to solve. For example, what are the most common side effects for all the medications prescribed for the current inpatients?

4. If you are a third-year nursing student ask to supervise a first- or second-year student in their orientation or with a specific care activity.

Summary

This chapter has explored the different people you will encounter and learn from in practice. The primary group to learn from are nurses. There are four developmental stages for nurses to support and assess students in practice. The key stage is Stage 2 – the mentor. The role of the mentor in terms of the mandatory requirements and responsibilities was presented along with examples of how to make best use of your time with your mentor.

A rationale was provided for students learning from service users and carers and the legalities of working with service users specifically in terms of the ethics of learning from service users and the importance of maintaining the rights of the service user. Working within a multidisciplinary team was acknowledged as another learning opportunity. The student was encouraged to identify from their own experience the different professions that make up the team. The theory of interprofessional learning was introduced with examples and the process of how it can be carried out using service user pathways and establishing clear learning outcomes.

Finally, the learning gained from peers was explored and the positive effects and new learning that can be achieved as a result of this approach were considered. A combined approach of learning from and with others – whether it is a nurse, service user, other professional or student – provides the most comprehensive real-time opportunity to maximise your learning in the CLE.

Knowledge review

See Appendix 5 to compare your answers.

1. How many developmental stages are there for nurses to support and assess students in practice?

2. What percentage of time must a mentor spend with you while giving direct care?

3. How will you integrate into a new team on each placement?

4. What are the protected characteristics?

5. What must you gain before any patient care?

6. What are the benefits of learning from service users/multidisciplinary team?

Further reading and resources

Centre for the Advancement of Interprofessional Education: https://www.caipe.org/resources

Person-centred care made simple: http://www.health.org.uk/sites/health/files/PersonCentredCareMadeSimple.pdf

Gillick competency test: https://www.nspcc.org.uk/preventing-abuse/child-protection-system/legal-definition-child-rights-law/gillick-competency-fraser-guidelines/

6

When?

Learning outcomes

After reading and completing the activities in this chapter you will be able to:

➤ Prepare for your placement.

➤ Examine the role of assessment to support learning.

➤ Utilise independent study time effectively.

So far in this book, you will have gained an appreciation as to why you learn in practice, recognised that the **clinical learning environment** (CLE) is where you learn and ascertained the numerous methods of how you can learn. Moreover, you will have determined what knowledge, skills and attitudes must be learnt, and differentiated between the separate groups of people who you can learn from.

This final chapter explores when you learn in practice by focusing on three key periods, namely the time before, during and after your placement. Before each placement you will have the opportunity to prepare for your learning in practice. Having identified the type of placement you have been allocated, you can begin to set your learning needs. During your placement you will then need to plan meetings with your mentor at the beginning, middle and end of the placement in order to initially tailor your learning opportunities and then on subsequent occasions review your progress.

A time often overlooked for learning is when you undertake your practice-based assessments. The principles of a fair assessment and the assessment process are explored. Linked to assessment is feedback and an explanation of how this supports your learning is included. Finally, during your placement your learning will occur over a 24/7 cycle and the practice of managing your learning in the face of varying shift patterns will be described.

The last section of the chapter looks at your learning after placement and the ongoing development of your knowledge, skills and attitudes. It will discuss the importance of utilising any allocated independent study time effectively and encourage you to apply the theory that you receive at university to the advancement of your nursing practice.

Before your placement

The allocation of your placement tends not to be your responsibility; however, it is worth establishing if you do have the option to choose or swop your placement. Your course will have administrators who form the placement team. These are university staff who are designated to arrange your placements. They will also most likely be responsible for maintaining the record of your completed hours and any absences – expected or otherwise. If you need to renegotiate your practice hours you would most likely need to seek approval from the course lead (see Activity 6.1 to help you identify key information about the allocation of your placements).

Activity 6.1 Understanding how your placements are arranged

Use the following questions as a prompt to help you understand the process of placement allocations.

- Review your course handbook – What information does it contain about placements?

- Where else is there information about placements?

- How are you notified about your placements?

- Who do you contact if you have queries about your allocated placement?

- Do you know the contact details of the placement team?

You may be made aware from when you start the course where all your placements will be for the whole of the three years. However, it can be difficult to issue each student with all their placement allocations in advance. More often than not you will be notified one placement at a time. The main reason for this is that the planning of placements is dependent on the availability and suitability of the clinical settings. Each placement must have a biannual audit and if this flags up issues these must be resolved before the placement can be used again. The constantly shifting landscape of practice means that what was perhaps an inpatient acute ward could in a year's time become an outpatient service. Therefore, predetermining placements will be subject to service reconfiguration and resourcing issues.

It is also probable that during your nursing education more clinical settings may become available and therefore you should not be disadvantaged from being able to access as wide a range of placements as possible. For example, if nursing staff subsequently become qualified **mentors** or **sign-off mentors** a practice area can become a placement. Within the private, voluntary and independent sector new clinical units, nursing homes, hospices and so on may emerge. Similarly, within the NHS innovative services are continually being developed that reflect the changing healthcare needs of the UK population, for example admission avoidance services, community intravenous therapy teams and integrated health and social care models.

Despite not knowing the specific hospital ward, GP surgery or respite centre that you may be allocated, your course will have planned your practice experiences according to a pathway. This may be published and made available to you with the proviso that it is subject to change or it may just be used by the university placement team to ensure that you experience a range of clinical settings over the three years. As a minimum the **Nursing and Midwifery Council** (NMC) require that you experience both hospital and community settings.

Tables 6.1, 6.2, 6.3 and 6.4 have examples for each nursing field of a placement pathway. The model used is to have three placements in each year. This may not be the model used on your course but it will give you an idea of the types of placements and when you are most likely to experience them. Community refers to community nursing, practice nurses, community hospital, intermediate care and so on. Day service refers to outpatients, day surgery, day medicine and so on. Specialist acute refers to theatres, emergency department, high dependency, critical care and so on. Specialist community refers to rapid access services, HIV and sexual health services, bladder and bowel services, minor injuries and so on. The final placement could be any one of the previously identified placement types, the only difference being that there would need to be access to a sign-off mentor in the placement.

The pathways may have repeated placement types, for example a medical ward is a placement both in year one and year three. This could be the exact same ward or a different medical ward. Both options have benefits: returning to the same ward would mean the student is familiar with the CLE and can review the development in their learning whereas a different ward would provide a new set of clinical experiences and learning opportunities. The difficulties of either approach would be if the student struggled in their previous placement due to poor mentoring, limited interest in the clinical speciality or other circumstances that restricted their learning, and with a new ward the student would have to familiarise themselves with a new team and new practices.

You will also note that the specialist clinical settings tend to be preserved for years two and three. This is because the complexity of the care and/or the acuity of the service will require a student to be more able to integrate within a team, to already have a good level of knowledge and skills in order to get the most out of the CLE and to be developing autonomous practice and the facility to work under indirect supervision. As a result, a year one student is not deemed to have sufficient exposure to and experience of healthcare in their role as a student nurse for the placement to be both beneficial and appropriate to their stage of learning.

Table 6.1 Example of a placement pathway for an Adult student nurse

Year 1	Year 2	Year 3
Medical ward	Day service	Surgical ward
Community	Specialist acute	Specialist community
Surgical ward	Community	Final placement

Table 6.2 Example of a placement pathway for a Children's nursing student nurse

Year 1	Year 2	Year 3
Community	Surgical ward	Medical ward
Medical ward	School nurse	Specialist community
Health Visitor	Specialist acute	Final placement

Table 6.3 Example of a placement pathway for a Learning Disabilities student nurse

Year 1	Year 2	Year 3
Respite	Learning Disability unit	Specialist community
Community	Residential care	Respite
School Nurse	Community	Final placement

Table 6.4   Example of a placement pathway for a Mental Health student
nurse

Year 1	Year 2	Year 3
Dementia care	Acute ward	Recovery
Recovery	Specialist community	Specialist acute
Community	Child and Adolescent	Final placement

Typically, you will receive notification in advance of your next allocated placement. This should ideally give you sufficient time to undertake
a period of focused preparation prior to starting. For a placement to be
successful, although somewhat of a cliché, it still remains true that 'failing to prepare means preparing to fail'. If there is material about the
placement, access this to help familiarise yourself with the type of placement you will be attending and to check what information the CLE gives
you about learning opportunities and what you will learn? This information is often presented in the form of a placement profile.

Placement profile

The majority of placement settings will have prepared a placement profile, intended for use by student nurses to read in advance of a placement
commencing. This information, which is generally found online, gives
you a clear understanding of the work of the area you have been allocated
to, the team you will be working within, and information that will support you while working in this area. It is common sense to take the time
to access and read in full this document to ensure that when you meet
with your mentor for the first time, you hold a clear understanding of the
remit of the department. Utilising your time in this way will also enable
you to prepare any questions in advance of the placement, so that you are
more likely to begin the learning experience as early into the start of the
placement as possible. Try Activity 6.2 to ensure you are making the most
of the placement profile.

Activity 6.2 Using the placement profile

Establish how and where the placement profiles are stored.

What level of detail do they contain?

▶

◀

How could the information contained in the profile help you prepare for your next placement?

- Are the contact details of the placement listed?
- Are the shift patterns listed?
- Is a nursing model used in the CLE?
- Are suggested learning experiences listed?
- Are members of the multidisciplinary team listed?

What else would you like to know about the placement?

If any of the details are incorrect who do you inform to get the profile updated?

Prior to starting you should also undertake a reflection on the knowledge, skills and attitudes that you have developed already and consider how these could be further enhanced in this new placement. It can also be helpful to review any action plans or feedback you have received from mentors in previous placements, as these will all help you to plan your learning needs. Again this reinforces the idea that placements are not to be viewed as isolated learning events; rather, they can be connected as you transfer and build upon previously acquired knowledge, skills and attitudes. You may also want to reflect on your feelings before going into the specific practice setting: What are you looking forward to? What concerns do you have and what actions do you need to take to resolve them?

Once you have been notified of the CLE you are heading to, it is best practice to make contact with the area to introduce yourself. Generally, a fortnight before should give you sufficient time to get through to the person you need to speak to and make the necessary arrangements in order for you to start at the appointed time. Depending on the location, you can either do this over the phone or in person. Bearing in mind the unpredictable nature of healthcare, you may opt to make the initial contact by phone, but you can always follow this up with an informal visit.

The purpose of this initial contact is to ensure that you are expected. (Rarely there may be an unexpected change in the circumstances of the clinical setting which could mean that the practice area is now unable to accommodate a student – learning of this well in advance would allow time for the placement team to arrange an alternate placement for you.) You can introduce yourself, establish the name of the mentor that will be supporting you while in the placement and agree the date on which you will start the first shift and the shift pattern for the first week at least.

Some placements, especially if they accommodate several students at a time, may wish for all new starters to come in on the same day so that a shared induction programme can be provided. During this initial conversation, you can also enquire as to how your shift pattern is managed, as some areas will allocate shifts to you, especially if they are busy and have a higher number of students in the department. Others may allow you to self-roster, with the condition that you have regular contact with your mentor or associate/buddy mentor.

Some clinical areas will have special requirements that you would need to adhere to, such as a non-standard uniform/specific dress code; and access arrangements (many settings, for example, have restricted access) may need to be made for you to be authorised with access to the department and to the information technology systems used for record keeping. In addition you may need to provide evidence of specific training such as breakaway, clearance with the disclosure and barring service (DBS), moving and handling, basic life support or provide evidence of compliance with guidelines to enable you to undertake independent visits to a service users home. See Box 6.1 for a summary of the recommendations to help you prepare for each placement.

Box 6.1 Key recommendations for preparing for a placement

- When contacting the placement for the first time, ask to speak with the nurse in charge. This person will be able to either help you straight away or know who you need to contact and when they will be available.

- Contact the placement in advance to establish who your mentor is and what your hours of working will be (at least for the first week).

- Identify any practicalities unique to that placement, for example security access and dress code.

- Plan your journey and how to find the placement in advance.

- Establish what to do in the event that you are late or you might be absent.

- Manage other commitments during your placement to ensure you are able to commit to the placement hours.

During your placement

Upon arrival in the designated placement, your learning can commence almost immediately. Therefore, it is important that you quickly feel settled and are ready to access the learning opportunities that are on offer.

To expedite this it is important that in the placement you meet formally with your mentor. The most common schedule is a minimum of three meetings, that is, a welcome meeting at the start, a progress review about halfway in to the placement and a summary meeting towards the end. The welcome meeting, which is typically held within the first few weeks, will be the first formal meeting with your mentor (and associate/buddy mentor). It is commonplace nowadays for a student to be allocated a primary mentor (who has overall responsibility for facilitating your learning) and a buddy or associate mentor.

The primary mentor must have undertaken and successfully completed an NMC-approved mentor preparation course, whereas the associate/buddy mentor may not yet have done so or may be in the process of completing the course. That said, you will also gain a great deal from working alongside all members of the clinical team (both registered professionals and support staff). As the NMC guidance states that you must work only 40% of the allocated placement time directly or indirectly under the supervision of your mentor, you should expect to work with many other people while on placement. Chapter 5 – 'Who?' – provides full details on the range of people within the CLE that you can learn from.

As part of your introductory meeting you will ideally set your **learning contract** which outlines the priorities and focus for your time on the placement. If the placement is to be successful, all parties (you and your mentor) need to be clear and in agreement about the expectations of the placement. You need to have a good working relationship with your mentor in order to feel comfortable in asking questions and seeking out learning opportunities. However, it is unreasonable to expect your mentor to be able to arrange assessments for all or the majority of your skills and competencies in a single placement. Many courses will require you to achieve and maintain specific skills and competencies in a particular academic year. Therefore, it would be prudent to have already identified these required assessments so that with each forthcoming placement you can determine which ones are suitable to work towards achieving.

Once the learning contract has been documented and agreed by you and your mentor, it is important to make time subsequently in the placement to review your progress. For a longer placement, it is sensible to agree a date with your mentor for a mid-point interview. As the name suggests, this is a review meeting approximately halfway through the placement that allows both parties to review your progress on the placement against the set learning contract, to make any necessary adjustments to keep you on track toward meeting all of your learning needs and to identify any new learning to be added. On occasions, you may need to amend or reprioritise certain activities in order to ensure that you gain the maximum benefit of your time in the CLE.

The final meeting is a summation of your learning and progress which again should be recorded in your **Assessment of Practice (AOP) document**. This will either confirm the completion of your learning contract or the development of an **action plan** to feed forward your learning for the next placement. At the completion of each placement, it is important for you as a learner to ensure that all relevant mandatory documentation is completed fully – and as an adult learner this responsibility falls to you personally and is not for your mentor to remember and organise. Try to schedule this final meeting with your mentor in the final few weeks of the placement – it is unwise to leave this meeting until the last day as it is inevitable that there will be circumstances outside of your control that will mean the meeting cannot happen. In the event contact your personal tutor to discuss how to resolve this.

As it is your responsibility to complete the AOP document and gather evidence of completion of the NMC competencies it is really important that you plan in advance your assessments and also the submission of the document to the agreed submission deadline. It may be that some sections are optional/formative and other sections are mandatory/summative. Read carefully and make sure you know what the requirements are and who needs to complete what. Simple omissions such as a date, name/ signature or confirmatory tick can mean a referral of the AOP document.

In addition to your mentor most placements now have a named individual who is responsible for the management of students while on placement. Typically, this would be a practice educator or a student coordinator. Chapter 3 – 'Where?' – provides more details on the specific support roles in practice. This person may have prepared a student welcome pack, which has information specific to the setting in which you are placed. It may contain a description of the type of care and services provided in this setting and abbreviations and common terms with definitions that you will come across. It may outline some of the skills and competencies that can be assessed and developed while you are on placement and it may provide examples of the varying learning opportunities available and the spoke experiences (see Chapter 2) that you could undertake.

As placements will be wide-ranging and diverse over the course of your nursing education it is not possible for you to receive a lecture on every aspect of clinical practice that you will encounter on placement. In addition, there will always be some areas of practice that you may feel more familiar with than others. It is reasonable and positively encouraged to

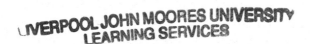

take the time while on placement to conduct a literature search and to access the library or local resources in the CLE to support your knowledge learning. For example, if you are allocated to a specialist ward, spend some time researching the commonly performed procedures that you are likely to encounter and the priorities in care for the service users. Or you may need to refresh your understanding of anatomy and physiology or pharmacology.

Assessment during your placement

If you are anything like the majority of students, you would probably prefer to just attend placement without having to worry about getting skills signed off. Some students even consider that the skills get in the way of really learning how to become a nurse. This does not mean assessment per se is wrong but the process of how an assessment is conducted in practice can be flawed. When do you really know you have learnt something? When you have completed an assessment and demonstrated the required learning outcomes. The value of assessment, therefore, is in confirming the extent of your learning and as a student on a professionally regulated course, assessment is the means of judging your professional competence, that is, am I safe and effective? It also gives you an awareness of the quality of your learning, that is, how well have I learnt how to be safe and effective?

There are two forms of assessment: formative and summative. The main difference being that formative assessment is the means of aiding learning, whereas summative assessment is the means of certifying the learning. Formative assessment is about participating in ongoing assessments so that by the time you get to your final (summative) assessment you are better prepared, having been able to act on the feedback you will have received from your mentor and other members of the clinical team. By regularly undertaking formative assessments it is hoped that you will be better prepared for the summative assessments as they will be less daunting and more familiar. Figure 6.1 shows this process mapped onto Kolb's experiential learning cycle.

Using a formative assessment as the concrete experience, the learner should undertake a reflective observation of the assessment to reflect how well they think they did. In the abstract conceptualisation stage the learner receives feedback from the assessor to help them make sense of their performance. Finally, the student, having applied their self-reflection, feedback and any resultant learning, undertakes a summative assessment as active experimentation to determine the level of learning achieved.

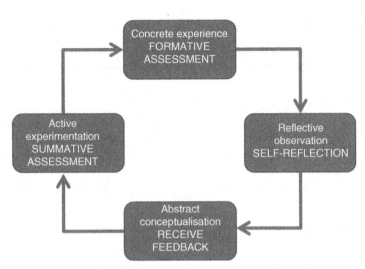

Figure 6.1 Diagram of assessment process mapped onto Kolb's experiential learning cycle

As a student on an undergraduate programme, each year of your course will have an agreed level of achievement with criteria which will define the complexity of the assessment and the knowledge, skills and attitudes expected of you. In each academic year, this criterion will increase the level of learning. So for example year one is assessed at level 4 (certificate), year two is assessed at level 5 (diploma) and year three (degree) is assessed at level 6. The scaling of the criteria starts at a basic level, but as you gain experience and progress through the course, the criteria is set at a higher level so that by the end of the course you should be demonstrating degree-level cognitive processes such as decision making, critical thinking and problem solving. Even if your practice-based assessments are pass/fail rather than graded they will still reflect the academic year of study and this progressive development in your knowledge, skills and attitudes.

There are nationally agreed descriptors for level 4–6 assessment criteria. The descriptors are grouped into five categories: setting; knowledge and understanding; cognitive skills; performance and practice; and personal and enabling skills. Each category is further subdivided with definitions of the nature of learning expected. Table 6.5 presents the five categories and subsections and Appendix 10 provides a comparative overview of the level 4, 5 and 6 descriptors according to each category.

Your AOP document will contain a list of the skills and NMC competencies that you will be expected to achieve in each and every year of the course. For each skill and competency there should be explicit criteria such as knowledge and practice descriptors (or the equivalent) which will outline what is expected from you and will form the basis of your

Table 6.5 The five categories for the descriptors of learning

Category	Subsection	Definition
Setting	Operational context	Where the learning takes place – therefore, by year three you will be expected to demonstrate your learning in more complex clinical settings.
	Autonomy and responsibility for actions	The autonomy exercised by the learner – therefore, by year three you would be expected to work more under indirect supervision.
Knowledge and understanding	Knowledge and understanding	The requisite knowledge and understanding – therefore, by year three you would be expected to have a greater knowledge base and understanding of nursing practice and the profession.
Cognitive skills	Conceptualisation and critical thinking	The appreciation of conceptual and abstract ideas – therefore, by year three you would be expected to question knowledge and practices to determine best practice.
	Problem solving research and enquiry	The undertaking of research and enquiry to solve problems – therefore, by year three you would be expected to determine the nature of a problem and the most appropriate means of enquiry to resolve it.
	Synthesis and creativity	The summation and use of your knowledge – therefore, by year three you would be expected to bring together your learning to innovatively provide care every time for every person.
	Analysis and evaluation	The weighing up of knowledge and information – therefore, by year three you would be expected to analyse the validity and acuity of data and findings to support clinical decision making.
Performance and practice	Adaption to context	Situational awareness of the context of practice and own knowledge/skill level – therefore, by year three you would be expected to apply knowledge to practice and make adaptions according to the environment and circumstances.
	Performance	Demonstration of skill – therefore, by year three you would be expected to carry out clinical and non-clinical skills safely and effectively.
	Team and organisational working	The facility to work with others and self-manage – therefore, by year three you would be expected to work well in teams and display time management and prioritisation of care.
	Ethical awareness and application	The awareness of taking an ethical approach – therefore, by year three you would be expected to work responsibly and work according to The Code (NMC 2015).

Personal and enabling skills	Personal evaluation and development	The awareness of self and strengths and weaknesses – therefore, by year three you would be expected to reflect and plan your learning and development needs.
	Interpersonal and communication skills	The skills required for effective interactions – therefore, by year three you would be expected to have the capability to communicate clearly and accurately, to interpret other's communications and show empathy, kindness and acceptance of others.

preparation for all forthcoming assessments. If you were to compare the terminology used in the document(s) at each level of assessment you will likely see a progression in the complexity and challenge. For example you may be required to define a concept at level 4 but then analyse and evaluate this concept at level 5 and finally synthesise this concept into your practice at level 6. This gradation should reassure you that you will not be expected to know everything on day one but rather the emphasis is on advancing you towards the goal of providing safe and effective care over the three years. To help you prepare for your assessments the remainder of this section will outline the principles of assessment.

Assessments should be valid

When you are assessed, although it is often not a pleasant experience to be observed and tested, you should at least be satisfied that it was fair. A valid assessment is one which measures what it is supposed to measure. If you are expected to demonstrate a particular skill, the assessment should be designed to test this, not any other. Having said that, it is difficult to separate out the skills and knowledge you need to be assessed on into discrete assessments. The best type of assessment, therefore, is one which does not just assess your ability in the current context but enables you to represent your learning and how you would apply it in related areas. For example, if you are being assessed on your communication skills when you conduct an admission interview, how well does this assessment predict your performance in areas such as a nursing handover or gaining consent?

To support a valid assessment you should first be made aware whether you are undertaking a formative or summative assessment and given time to prepare. Ideally, you should also take the opportunity to work through the assessment criteria with your assessor. Hopefully the criteria you are assessed against is clear but it may still lack sufficient detail. If you were asked to list the main risk factors of a disease or condition how many would you need to give to know you have provided the main ones? Having a conversation before you are assessed will mean that you and your assessor will be familiar with the assessment, you will understand what is expected of you and you will be in agreement about how you will demonstrate this criteria, that is, which assessment strategy will be employed.

Finally, you need to determine if you are fit to complete the assessment. Are their circumstances that are impacting on your ability to perform at your best? Again discuss these with your mentor and also your personal tutor as you may need to defer an assessment and seek further support before you attempt an assessment and then unduly fail.

Assessments should be reliable

Regrettably, you will have variable experiences of being assessed by mentors. Some will be very particular and thorough; others will adopt a casual and less methodical approach. While on the surface your preferred option may be to have a 'light' assessment the consequences are such that the extent of your preparation will not be acknowledged, the depth and breadth of your learning will not be fully assessed and you may remain unaware of any gaps in your learning or any errors that will be perpetuated. The assessor role is about creating as relaxed an atmosphere as possible, respecting the effort and preparation you have put in, giving you the opportunity to perform to the best of your capability and applying their professional judgement while following the assessment criteria when making their decision.

Taylor's story (Adult nursing student)

'The thing we talked about most was how our assessments in practice were so different, depending on where we were and who was assessing us. It was the most frustrating when you prepare for an assessment and the mentor just asks a few questions and signs you off. You kind of need a bit more testing to make sure you really do know and understand everything.'

The most reliable assessment is one which produces the same results regardless of the assessor or the person being assessed, that is, there is a consistency about the assessment such that if the assessment was carried out by a different assessor they would reach the same conclusion.

Reliability in assessment, therefore, is about removing subjectivity and remaining objective. Again using the assessment criteria as the standard against which you are assessed reduces the likelihood of subjectivity creeping into the assessment.

A key variable in your practice-based assessments is the practice area itself. The assessment may have to be postponed because of changing clinical priorities, the assessment may become more complex than anticipated due to alterations in the patient's condition, or it may be that the environment is just simply too distracting. You would not undertake a written exam in the middle of a ward environment but somehow you are still expected to complete an assessment in this busy, fluctuant setting. Participating in formative assessments can help you manage your responses to the environment and anticipate possible distractions.

Liz's story (Children's nursing student)

'I often prepare for assessments by putting myself in the shoes of the patient. Do I feel that the person in front of me knows what they are talking about and demonstrates a safe level of practice?'

Assessment strategies

There are a number of ways in which you will be assessed; the most common is through direct observation. This is where your mentor will sample your performance on a given day at a given time. This highlights the distinction between skills and competency assessments. The skills that you will be required to achieve are snapshots of your knowledge, skills and attitudes completed on an agreed day and time. The NMC competencies, however, are an overview of your achievement over the entirety of the placement. As a result, the competencies tend to be 'signed off' towards the end of the placement once your mentor has had sufficient time to observe and gather feedback from others about your behaviour and performance throughout the placement.

Questioning will be another frequently used assessment method. Chapter 3 – 'How?' – explored the use of questioning in your learning but you should also expect your assessor to ask you questions as part of an assessment. As a result you should agree when you would find it easiest to answer these questions, that is, perhaps not during the practical element of an assessment. The questions will establish your knowledge but should also examine your reasoning and evaluative skills. A helpful approach to take when providing your answers is to link your answer to a service user. This will make it more relevant and applied rather than just a list of abstract ideas and concepts. For example, if you were asked to name and talk about some infection prevention and control strategies, you could give an example of a time when you applied these measures in the care of a particular patient – for example, in the case of hand hygiene before and after care giving you may also have needed to wear personal protective equipment; you could then also talk through safe disposal of waste and so on. If you have not provided all of the strategies your mentor can then simply ask you 'What else?' to allow you to complete the answer. Box 6.2 lists other formative and summative assessment strategies that you may encounter or request in your practice-based assessments.

Box 6.2 Practice-based assessment strategies

Direct observation

Questioning

Reflective discussion

Presentation

Simulation

Reflective writing

Self-assessment

There may be occasions when you may not meet the standard required to pass an assessment. In such an event measures should be put in place to highlight and address the deficit(s) and be recorded in an action plan devised to support you for reattempt at the assessment. If you are experiencing difficulty over a range of skills or NMC competencies your mentor has a duty to discuss such concerns with your personal tutor to enable suitable learning support to be put in place.

An ongoing concern with assessment in nursing education is that assessment processes are not robust and there is a tendency among many mentors of a 'failure to fail'. This trend of passing students when they should be failed was first reported by Kathleen Duffy in 1994. She identified that mentors would give the student the benefit of the doubt if there was any question as to the ability of the student's performance (Duffy 1994). If poor performance and knowledge on the part of the student remains unchallenged the logical outcome is that this student becomes a registered nurse who is neither safe nor effective. You should be prepared that if your mentor has any concerns about your capabilities as a nurse, they will raise these with you in the first instance, and then in conjunction with your mentor you will work towards addressing the shortfall. Ultimately, your mentor has a duty to both protect the welfare of the service users and to safeguard the reputation of the nursing profession.

Feedback during your placement

Throughout the placement you will receive feedback on your learning. This may be informal – for example, when you receive comments from your mentor, another practitioner or a service user about your nursing care. On other occasions you may seek more formal feedback from your mentor on your progress. Similarly, you will receive feedback following an assessment. Generally, it is this feedback from your mentors that is used as the main source of guidance on how well you are performing and progressing. The latter two types of feedback should begin with a self-assessment of your development followed by a constructive discussion of your strengths and weaknesses. Most importantly, you should use the AOP document as a way to capture this feedback. Often provision is made within the AOP document of specific feedback sections to be completed during and at the end of each placement. The feedback may also be subsumed within the development of an action plan. See Chapter 4 – 'What?' – for more details on how to devise an action plan. Box 6.3 has an example of a student's feedback written in their AOP document.

Box 6.3 Example of student feedback

During this placement I have tried out different communication methods with people with dementia and recognise the value of non-verbal communication. I have been able to establish and maintain a therapeutic relationship with service users and it has been really satisfying to know that they trust me and feel comfortable when I care for them. I am aware of my limitations and the importance of liaising with the multidisciplinary team.

So far I have achieved three of my learning outcomes from my learning contract and I am organising a departmental visit to help achieve a further learning need to understand the admissions process better. I would like to work on my knowledge of medication and also build my confidence in giving a handover to a nurse.

Completing your practice hours

You will need to consult the specific requirements of your course, but most programmes will expect that at some point over the three years you gain experience of the full period of 24/7 shift patterns. This will therefore include you having to work night shifts, weekends and bank holidays. The clinical, and therefore your learning, experiences will be very different in what is regularly referred to as 'out of hours' working. The intensity of the work may be less, although this is not an absolute and is very much dependent on the clinical setting. Access to ancillary services such as pathology, pharmacy, catering and so on may only be available via an on-call service and the pattern of working will be dictated by the requirement to preserve the normal sleep/wake cycle of the service users, to limit procedures that would require senior overview but are carried out by less experienced juniors and to maintain continuity of the service on reduced staffing numbers and clinical mix.

It is important that you recognise the demands on you and the distinctions in working different shift patterns in terms of both your learning and your physical and mental well-being. Many clinical areas have adopted a long-day system whereby staff complete a shift from morning to evening rather than either an early or late shift. The long day shift is a minimum of 12 hours rather than 7.5 hours. Students have varying responses to this shift pattern but it is important to remember that, regardless of your preference, as you are supernumerary you do not necessarily have to follow the precise shift pattern of the CLE.

Rachel's story (Adult nursing student)

'I was cleared as fit for practice by occ health but with my chronic health condition I found that I was really struggling with the long days. I would end up being sick and missing placement. I asked the university to review my learning support plan and I had it stipulated that I should work the normal 7.5 hours rather than 12.5. This made a real difference, I was having to go into placement more frequently but for less time which helped with continuity and my general health as I felt less exhausted and I didn't need to recover after each shift.'

Joshua's story (Mental Health nursing student)

'It took me a while to get used to the shift patterns. The days can be very long and if you add on the travel time either end of the day it is pretty full on.'

You may need to question your motivation if your only reason for working long days is simply so that you spend less time in practice throughout the week. Nevertheless, as you will encounter the long-day system as a registered nurse it is helpful now as a student to learn how to manage the demands of working 12 hours especially if you work two or even three long days in a row. Even simple things like bringing sufficient meals or money to buy food and arranging your time can maintain a good work–life balance. The time when you will definitely have to work 12 hours will be on a night shift. Although some clinical areas may have twilights where you start in the evening and finish in the early part of the night shift, for example 6 p.m. to 11 p.m. Box 6.4 has some top tips to help you prepare and manage working on a night shift.

Box 6.4 Top tips for surviving a night shift

- A night shift does not mean you have a full working day before: try to rest rather than cram lots of things in.

- Ask friends and family to be positive about night shifts. It is even harder if all you hear people saying is, '*I could never do a night shift*' or '*I would hate to do a night shift.*'

- Take warm clothing as you are likely to feel cold in the early hours of the morning. (Research why you feel cold at about 4 a.m. in the morning!)

- Decide when and how much you want to eat before, during and after the night shift. (This will be trial and error; some people completely reverse their meals, that is, have breakfast the evening before and dinner the morning after; other people stick to regular meals, some snack/eat a meal(s) during the shift and other people avoid eating anything at all.)

- Keep well-hydrated during the night shift.

- Associated with your eating and drinking be aware of 'night wind'! As your digesting and resting patterns will be out of sync you may experience bloating and trapped wind.

- Ask your mentor how they prepare for a night shift.

- Decide with your mentor what learning you will achieve; nights are often a great time to bond with colleagues, ask questions and review your knowledge.

- Be safe; if you are too tired to drive take an alternative means of transport home.

- Invest in eye shades and earplugs to help you sleep during the day.

- Tell people you are sleeping after a night shift and not to disturb you; switch your phone to silent.

A condition of your learning support plan may be that you only work short shifts, that is, 7.5 hours and/or your total weekly practice hours may be reduced to accommodate your personal circumstances. Your mentor will understandably expect you to have at least some experience of starting or finishing at the times of shift handovers. This will enable you to develop the skills of handover and assessing and prioritising care needs. Even without a learning support plan, many students and mentors recommend working only early and/or late shifts. It is important to not underestimate the concentration and effort required on the part of both your mentor and you to facilitate your learning over an extended period of time. The drawbacks of working long days, which will impact on your learning, include increased levels of tiredness and stress, safety issues (reduced concentration, making more mistakes, ineffective communication and poor teamwork) and the increased health risks (depressive states, anxiety, sleep disturbance, heart disease) (Skills for Care 2015).

The importance of meeting the specified total of practice hours (2300 hours) over the duration of the course means your university will have a system for recording your attendance on placement. Some systems may be electronic; others may be paper-based and require you to obtain a signature from your mentor to verify attendance on any given shift. Irrespective of the system, do ensure that you are familiar and comply with the process applicable to you. Likewise, if you are unwell during a placement and are unable to attend, treat the setting exactly the same as if you were at work and make contact by telephone in advance of the start of the shift to notify your mentor or the departmental lead of your absence. In most cases, universities will expect you to follow this up with a call to the school office so that internal records may be updated. If your absence is to be ongoing, it is only courtesy to keep your placement area informed.

After your placement

After your placement you should reflect on the overall experience you have had and identify key learning you need to follow up in subsequent placements. If you have been referred in any assessments while on placement, your mentor should have created an action plan for you to follow in the next placement.

Most universities and practice areas will ask you to complete a placement evaluation questionnaire. This is generally optional, though strongly encouraged, as it allows mentors and placements to see what they are doing well and understand where they can improve the CLE for future students. The evaluation is also a good opportunity to aid your personal reflections. You can give consideration to the key learning opportunities experienced, as well as areas that could have been explored in more depth.

When back in university, look to consolidate your experience of practice by:

➤ relating the taught content to what you have seen on placement

➤ contributing to group discussions as this will help affirm your understanding

➤ incorporating your practice experiences into academic assignments, for example case studies and reflective accounts.

For many students, sessions such as problem-, enquiry- or experienced-based learning (see the 'Further reading and resources' section below) are useful learning strategies for making sense of any areas of practice that have been problematic. It is of course worth remembering that your personal tutor is always available for you to discuss any concerns you may have about practice or to clarify your learning gained in practice.

Finally, be mindful of any practical requirements that you should complete once the placement has ended – for example, do you have a specialised uniform that belongs to the department that you need to return? Have you been allocated a locker that needs to be emptied? It is also wise to thank the placement for the experience provided to you; after all, in years to come these people may well be your employer and it is prudent to bear in mind that a good reputation as a student could serve you well when it comes to entering the job market for the first time.

Independent study

From a quick glance at your timetable you will undoubtedly be able to identify several hours allocated to 'independent study' or guided reading. While it may be tempting to view this as free time, or an opportunity to take time away from the course, do not underestimate the importance and significance of such study allocations. Undoubtedly, as an adult learner you will be fulfilling the need for ongoing study by consolidating your prior learning and preparing for new learning in practice through independent study. If you have allocated independent study time it is worthwhile finding out if the skills room facilities on the university campus can be accessed for additional practice time (supervised or unsupervised).

After your placement the cycle will recommence once again as you prepare for your next placement. However, the intention with each new placement is that what you hope to achieve (based upon your reflections, feedback and action plans) will be moving you closer to your goal of safe and effective practice.

Summary

This final chapter has focused on when you learn in practice, specifically in relation to the time before, during and after your placement. The time before your placement is critical as once you have received information about your allocated placement the process of preparing and contacting the placement can begin.

The second time frame is during the placement within which your time can be further divided into the start, the middle and the end. Other chapters have reviewed how and what you learn and this chapter has explored *when* your learning is confirmed, which is through assessment. Students should be entitled to fair – meaning valid and reliable – assessments. Concomitant with assessments is feedback and the mechanisms of receiving informal and formal feedback were presented. A consideration of when you learn also incorporated a review of the practical elements of completing the required NMC hours, such as how to manage working the different shift patterns including nights and long days.

The final time period is when you learn after the placement. Learning strategies were suggested such as reflection, reviewing your written feedback and any action plans recorded in the AOP document. When you return to university, you should expect to apply your practice learning in your academic study through both your contributions in scheduled sessions and your reference to your practice experiences in your module assignments. Finally, you looked at how your allocated independent study time can be put to effective use by consolidating your understanding of what you have learnt in practice and preparing for the next placement.

Knowledge review

See Appendix 6 to compare your answers.

1. In what ways could more clinical settings become available over the course of your nursing education?

2. What is a placement profile?

3. What are the two forms of assessment and how are they different?

4. What are some recommendations to support working a night shift?

5. How can independent study support your practice learning?

Further reading and resources

SEEC descriptors full document: http://www.seec.org.uk/wp-content/
    uploads/2016/07/SEEC-descriptors-2016.pdf
Problem-based learning: http://www.ceebl.manchester.ac.uk/ebl/

Glossary

Action plan: a written plan with detailed actions to be completed in order to achieve specified learning outcomes.

Activities of daily living: routine activities that people tend to do every day without needing assistance, such as eating, bathing, dressing, toileting, walking.

Adult learning: based on the idea that adults learn differently to children, and that adults have the capacity to be more self-directed and plan their own learning.

Assessment of Practice (AOP) document: this is the evidence of your achievement of the assessments that you undertake in practice. It may be a hard copy or electronic and may cover all three years or each year separately. Alternative terms include practice assessment document (PAD), clinical skills book, ongoing record of achievement (ORA) and practice portfolio.

Best practice: procedures that are accepted as being correct or most effective according to the latest available evidence.

Clinical learning environment (CLE): refers to the varying practice settings that student nurses will have allocated to them as *placements*.

Competency framework: the outline of the requirements that student nurses must meet in order to join the professional nursing register.

Compliant: the extent to which the service user's behaviour matches the clinician's recommendations for treatment and care.

Concordant: agreement between the clinician and the service user about the therapeutic decisions in the care of the service user.

Conflict resolution training: the means of providing people with the skills to spot signs of a potentially violent incident before it escalates. It teaches them how to defuse, prevent and manage an incident without the use of physical restraint. These skills are a safe and more ethical way to prevent an incident of violence. Physical restraint must be the last resort.

Continuous Professional Development (CPD): describes the learning activities professionals engage in to develop and enhance their knowledge, skills and attitudes in their profession. This may include academic study, revalidation, specialist education and mandatory training.

Cultural sensitivity: having an awareness of similarities and differences in culture and how this impacts on nursing care. Culture should be understood in its broadest sense rather than as a geographical determinant.

Curriculum: the subjects or content making up a programme of study. This can be locally agreed or determined by national or legislative requirements. The curriculum may be established and reviewed by professionals and regulatory bodies.

Essential skills clusters (ESC): support the achievement of the NMC competencies by identifying a range of essential skills common to all fields of nursing.

Ethical practice: relates to 'right' and 'wrong' conduct.

Evidence-based practice (EBP): the integration of clinical knowledge, values and the best available research evidence into the decision making process for the care of service users.

Experiential learning: a learning theory developed by Kolb based on the premise that learning occurs from reflection on experiences.

Higher education: the name given to study at university and the attainment of a higher qualification such as a diploma, degree, masters or PhD.

Higher education institute (HEI): any university that provides education and research facilities for undergraduate and postgraduate students. It is the highest level of education after school and further education/college.

Hub and spoke model: in this model each individual placement acts as 'the hub' which then has conjoined 'spoke' experiences of varying number and practice settings.

Human factors: encompass all those factors that can influence people and their behaviour. In a work context, human factors are the environmental, organisational and job factors, and individual characteristics which influence behaviour at work.

Human rights: human rights are the basic rights and freedoms that belong to every person in the world. In the UK human rights are protected by the *Human Rights Act 1998*.

Human Rights Act 1998: the Human Rights Act is a UK law passed in 1998. It means that you can defend your rights in the UK courts and that public organisations (including the Government, the Police and local councils) must treat everyone equally, with fairness, dignity and respect.

International Council of Nurses (ICN): is an alliance of more than 130 national nurse associations representing more than 16 million nurses worldwide. The ICN works to support quality nursing care for all, to ensure sound global health policies, to advance nursing knowledge and to sustain a respected, competent and satisfied nursing workforce.

Learning contract: is an individualised agreement between you and your mentor, of your learning needs.

Long-term conditions: long-term conditions or chronic diseases are conditions for which there is currently no cure, and are managed with drugs and other treatment, for example diabetes, depression, arthritis, asthma, epilepsy, hypertension, personality disorders.

Mentor: a registered nurse who, following successful completion of an NMC-approved mentor preparation programme, facilitates the learning and assessment of a student nurse while in practice.

Morally aware: means being aware of your own or the profession's principles regarding what is deemed as right and wrong.

National Health Service (NHS): the UK's publicly funded healthcare system. It is based on the principle established in the Health Services Act (1948) of care free at the point of delivery.

NMC Code (2015): sets out the required professional standards and behaviours expected of registered nurses and midwives. As a student you will also be expected to adhere to these.

Nursing and Midwifery Council (NMC): the governing body for nurses and midwives in the UK.

Nursing and Midwifery Order 2001: establishes the NMC: sets out the primary purpose of protecting the public, the structure of the organisation and its functions and activities.

Nursing field: nursing fields identify the specific individuals/populations that the nurse is registered to care for. The four fields are adult, children's, learning disabilities and mental health. All fields have generic and specific competencies.

Patient safety: can be described in terms of optimising processes, minimising risk and maximising efficient, accurate performance.

Placement: an allocated area of clinical practice that a student nurse will spend a designated period of time in, in order to achieve their practice learning and assessments.

Placement profile: published information about the placement including staff contact details, a description of the healthcare activities undertaken in the clinical area and the available learning opportunities.

Preceptorship: a structured period of transition for newly registered nurse, when they start their first employee position.

Professional, Statutory and Regulatory Body (PSRB): describes organisations (such as the NMC) which are authorised to accredit, approve or recognise specific programmes in HEIs in the context of professional requirements.

Progression points: separate the nursing programme into three equal parts: the first progression point is normally at the end of year one and the second progression point is normally at the end of year two. Progression on the course is subject to acquiring the minimum level of competence assigned to each progression point.

Reasonable adjustments: modifications made to a student's time and activity on placement to better support their learning in practice.

Reflection: the action of engaging in thinking about an experience and seeking to understand this better in order to support learning and growth (personal and professional).

Resilience: the ability to overcome adversity or difficulties.

Safeguarding: means protecting people's health, well-being and human rights, and enabling them to live free from harm, abuse and neglect.

Service user: a person who is a patient or other user of health and/or social services.

Sign-off mentor: a mentor who has undergone further assessments in order to be able to consider the practice evidence in the final placement to make a judgement that all competencies have been met and that the student is considered proficient and able to join the professional register.

Simulation: high or low fidelity replication of clinical scenarios to test out knowledge, skills and attitudes.

Spoke experience: a learning experience that is supplementary to the learning gained through a placement.

Situational awareness: the ability to see the bigger picture. During a crisis staff need to be able to appreciate alternative methods or the availability of other resources.

Supernumerary: means that the student will not, as part of their programme of preparation, be contracted by any person or body to provide nursing care.

Sustainability: means meeting our current needs without compromising the ability of future generations to meet their own needs.

Unconscious bias: an unintentional response to situational cues, for example a person's skin colour or accent that unknowingly influences a person's perception and behaviour towards others.

World Health Organization (WHO): is recognised as the authority on international health within the United Nation's member states.

Appendix 1 – Chapter 1 knowledge review answers

1. **What are the benefits to the learner of completing higher education?**

   ➤ *raised level of self-awareness*

   ➤ *critical thinking*

   ➤ *problem solving*

   ➤ *knowledge of cultures*

   ➤ *tolerance and acceptance of diversity*

2. **What is an appropriate term to describe a key attribute of an adult learner?**
   Self-directed.

3. **What document must all nursing programmes in the UK adhere to?**
   NMC Standards for Pre-registration Nursing Education (NMC 2010).

4. **How many theory and practice hours comprise a UK nursing course?**
   2300 theory, 2300 practice.

5. **What are some of the unique elements/advantages of learning in practice?**

   ➤ *emersion in practice*

   ➤ *development of role identity*

   ➤ *assessment of practice*

   ➤ *direct contact with patients*

Appendix 2 – Chapter 2 knowledge review answers

1. **What are the prerequisites for a CLE?**
   A safe and supportive environment and a quality-assured placement.

2. **Which placement types are present in all healthcare sectors – NHS, private and independent?**

   ➣ *assisted living*

   ➣ *residential care*

   ➣ *nursing home*

3. **How would you define experiential learning?**
   By experiencing practice you will participate in interactions with the environment, people and tasks. These experiences may or may not fit with your current knowledge level and ability. By reflecting on these experiences you can go on to construct greater knowledge and skills and a more meaningful understanding of yourself as a learner and your nursing practice. According to Kolb in order for this learning to happen the learner should move through a four-stage cycle – concrete experience, reflective observation, abstract conceptualisation and active experimentation.

4. **How often should you provide best practice as a student nurse and once registered?**
   Every time to every service user.

Appendix 3 – Chapter 3 knowledge review answers

1. **What examples can you give of building up your resilience?**

   - *build positive beliefs in your abilities*
   - *develop a strong social network*
   - *embrace change*
   - *be optimistic*
   - *nurture yourself*
   - *develop your problem-solving skills*
   - *establish goals*
   - *keep working on your abilities and qualities*

2. **What are the benefits to you knowing your learning style?**

   - *you will be able to increase your awareness of how you learn which will lead to improvements in your learning*
   - *you will be better able to make your learning style fit learning opportunities*
   - *you will be able to strengthen weaker learning styles*
   - *you will be better able to overcome difficulties encountered with your learning*
   - *you will be better able to manage your mentor's style of teaching*

3. **What are the four learning styles and how are they defined according to Honey and Mumford?**

Activist	• Activists learn by experience
	• Activist require an open mind
	• Activists prefer to involve themselves fully in experiences
Theorist	• Theorists learn by understanding the theory behind the experience
	• Theorists require information about the experience
	• Theorists prefer to analyse and synthesise experiences
Pragmatist	• Pragmatists learn by testing out learning on new experiences
	• Pragmatists require concrete rather than abstract examples/experiences
	• Pragmatists prefer time to process learning experiences
Reflector	• Reflectors learn by observing and thinking about experiences
	• Reflectors require distance from the experience
	• Reflectors prefer to view the experience from different perspectives

4. **What are the four broad learning strategies?**

   1. Exposure to an experience

   2. Participation in an experience

   3. Reflection on an experience

   4. Reinforcement of an experience

Appendix 4 – Chapter 4 knowledge review answers

1. **What is a learning contract?**
   A learning contract is an individualised agreement between you and your mentor of your learning needs.

2. **What is the difference between a learning contact and an action plan?**
   Action plans are a means of feeding forward your learning in to your next placement. Whereas a learning contract is speculative – that is, it contains what you hope to learn/achieve in the placement – an action plan is definitive – it will contain precise learning needs that may be outstanding from the learning contract or newly identified learning needs.

3. **What is a metaparadigm and what are the four specific metaparadigms in nursing?**
   A metaparadigm is basically the overarching view of a profession or discipline. It identifies what concepts are of interest to the discipline and the relationships that exist between these concepts. The agreed theory of nursing is based on Lee and Fawcett's work from 1978 which defined four metaparadigms central to nursing, namely the human being, nursing, health and the environment.

4. **Which section of The Code refers to delegation?**
   Section 11.

5. **Name the human factors and non-technical skills related to healthcare.**
   Human factors

   ➤ *workload demands*

   ➤ *physical/mental demands of the task*

   ➤ *the design of a device/product*

   ➤ *the process of the task*

   ➤ *the physical environment*

Non-technical skills

➤ *communication*

➤ *teamwork*

➤ *leadership*

➤ *decision making*

➤ *time management*

➤ *situational awareness*

➤ *values and beliefs*

6. **What term has superseded 'patient-centred' care?**
Person-centred care.

Appendix 5 – Chapter 5 knowledge review answers

1. **How many developmental stages are there for nurses to support and assess students in practice?**
   Four.

2. **What percentage of time must a mentor spend with you whilst giving direct care?**
   While giving direct care at least 40% of a student's time must be spent being supervised (directly or indirectly) by a mentor.

3. **How will you integrate into a new team in each placement?**
   Be familiar with the structure and purpose of the team, be authentic in your interactions with team members, be realistic about being a team member and be supportive of the team.

4. **What are the protected characteristics?**
   Age, disability, gender reassignment, pregnancy and maternity (which includes breastfeeding), race, religion or belief, sex and sexual orientation.

5. **What must you gain before any patient care?**
   Consent.

6. **What are the benefits of learning from service users/multidisciplinary team?**
   Service user – you will get to know yourself better, the level of your knowledge and skills, your professionalism, your resilience and your ability to respond appropriately to patients; you will learn how to personalise the care that you provide; the care of a person also will challenge your assumptions and stereotypes enabling you to develop a non-judgemental and open approach to caring for people.

   MDT – sharing of teaching and learning resources, increasing a culture of awareness and respect of each profession. Improved communication and working relationships. Addressing stereotyping and increased appreciation of each other's priorities, demands.

Appendix 6 – Chapter 6 knowledge review answers

1. **In what ways could more clinical settings become available over the course of your nursing education?**

   ➤ *If nursing staff subsequently become qualified mentors or sign-off mentors and the placement receives a successful audit.*

   ➤ *If within the private, voluntary and independent sector new clinical units, nursing homes, hospices and so on may emerge.*

   ➤ *If within the NHS innovative services are developed, for example admission avoidance services, community intravenous therapy teams, integrated health and social care models.*

2. **What is a placement profile?**
   This is information, which is generally found online, that gives you a clear understanding of the work of the area you have been allocated to, the team you will be working within and information that will support you while working in this area.

3. **What are the two forms of assessment and how are they different?**
   There are two forms of assessment: formative and summative. The main difference being formative assessment is the means of aiding learning whereas summative assessment is the means of certifying the learning.

4. **What are some recommendations to support working a night shift?**

   ➤ *A night shift does not mean you have a full working day before: try to rest rather than cram lots of things in.*

   ➤ *Ask friends and family to be positive about night shifts.*

   ➤ *Take warm clothing as you are likely to feel cold in the early hours of the morning.*

   ➤ *Decide when and how much you want to eat before, during and after the night shift.*

➤ *Keep well-hydrated during the night shift.*

➤ *Ask your mentor how they prepare for a night shift.*

➤ *Decide with your mentor what learning you will achieve.*

➤ *Be safe; if you are too tired to drive take an alternative means of transport home.*

➤ *Invest in eye shades and earplugs to help you sleep during the day.*

➤ *Tell people you are sleeping after a night shift and not to disturb you; switch your phone to silent.*

5. **How can independent study support your practice learning?**

➤ *It can help you consolidate your learning.*

➤ *It can help you understand areas of clinical practice that you may not fully comprehend.*

➤ *It can help you prepare for your next placement.*

Appendix 7 – Mindfulness exercise

Mindfulness is about being alert and accepting the experience of being in the moment rather than focusing on the past or the future. It is not about letting your mind go blank but stilling yourself and being aware of sensations and thoughts as they arise. It is about being aware of your responses to these sensations and thoughts and challenging these responses so you may be able to respond in a more constructive way.

Use your breathing as a focus point to remain in the present and keep your attention.

Five-minute mindfulness exercise

➢ Get comfortable on a chair; you can close your eyes if you like.

➢ Notice how your body is feeling and any physical movements.

➢ Notice any thoughts or feelings that you may have. Acknowledge these and let them go if they take you out of being in the moment.

➢ Now bring your attention to your breathing.

➢ Stay with your breathing in and out for 1 minute.

➢ Consider the following statement – *'You are not so concerned about the future with its thoughts and feelings, you are more aware of the present.'*

➢ If you get distracted or your mind wanders bring yourself back to your breathing and count 10 breaths in a row and then return to the statement.

➢ Gently return to the present.

Appendix 8 – Reflective questions

What was most familiar/different about the experience?

Is there any pattern that you can recognise in the experience?

What was the most/least fulfilling part of the experience?

What, if anything, happened that contradicted your prior knowledge, skills and attitude?

How do you feel about the experience now compared with how you felt about it at the time?

What does the experience suggest to you about your strengths/weaknesses?

What was more/less successful than you anticipated about the experience?

What might you do differently as a result of the experience?

What actions do your reflections lead you to?

Appendix 9 – Strengths, Weaknesses, Opportunities and Threats (SWOT) analysis tool

Using the SWOT analysis tool will help you identify your learning needs and the potential problems and how these can be addressed to achieve your learning needs. A template with prompt questions is provided below:

Strengths	Weaknesses
What are your successes in learning?	What are your difficulties in learning?
What have you achieved so far?	What have you not achieved so far?
•	•
•	•
•	•
Opportunities	**Threats**
Who or what is available to support your learning?	Who or what may limit your learning?
What motivates your learning?	What demotivates your learning?
•	•
•	•
•	

Use the strengths to take advantage of the opportunities.

Use the strengths to overcome weaknesses.

Use the opportunities to minimise threats.

Appendix 10 – Comparison of level 4, 5 and 6 descriptors

Acknowledgment: SEEC (2016) credit level descriptors for Higher Education available at www.seec.org.uk

Category	Level 4	Level 5	Level 6
Setting			
Operational context	Operates in a range of varied but predictable context that require the use of a specified range of techniques and information sources.	Operates in situations of varying complexity and predictability requiring the application of a wide range of techniques and information sources.	Operates in complex and unpredictable contexts, requiring selection and application from a range of largely standard techniques and information sources.
Autonomy and responsibility for actions	Acts with limited autonomy, under direction or supervision, within defined guidelines. Takes responsibility for the nature and quality of outputs.	Acts with limited supervision and direction within defined guidelines, accepting responsibility for achieving personal and/or group outcomes and/or outputs.	Acts with minimal supervision or direction within agreed guidelines, taking responsibility for accessing support and accepting accountability for determining and achieving personal and/or group outcomes.

Knowledge and understanding

	Level 4	Level 5	Level 6
Knowledge and understanding	Has a broad understanding of the knowledge base and its terminology or discourse. Appreciates that areas of this knowledge base are open to ongoing debate and reformulation.	Has detailed knowledge of well-established theories and concepts. Demonstrates an awareness of different ideas, contexts and frameworks and recognises those areas where the knowledge base is most/least secure.	Has a systematic understanding of the knowledge base and its inter-relationship with other fields of study. Demonstrates current understanding of some specialist areas in depth.

Cognitive skills

	Level 4	Level 5	Level 6
Conceptualisation and critical thinking	Identifies principles and concepts underlying theoretical frameworks and approaches, identifying their strengths and weaknesses.	Identifies, analyses and communicates principles and concepts, recognising competing perspectives.	Works with ideas at a level of abstraction, arguing from competing perspectives. Identifies the possibility of new concepts within existing knowledge frameworks and approaches.
Problem solving, research and enquiry	Identifies a well-defined focus for enquiry, plans and undertakes investigative strategies using a limited and defined range of methods, collects data from a variety of sources, and communicates results effectively in an appropriate format.	Undertakes research to provide new information and/or explores new or existing data to identify patterns and relationships. Uses appropriate theoretical models to judge the significance of the data collected, recognising the limitations of the enquiry.	Demonstrates confidence and flexibility in identifying and defining complex problems. Identifies, selects and uses investigative strategies and techniques to undertake a critical analysis, evaluating the outcomes.
Synthesis and creativity	Collects information from a variety of authoritative sources to inform a choice of solutions to standard problems in familiar contexts.	Collects and synthesises information to inform a choice of solutions to problems in unfamiliar contexts.	Applies knowledge in unfamiliar contexts, synthesising ideas or information to generate novel solutions. Achieves a body of work or practice that is coherent and resolved.

	Level 4	Level 5	Level 6
Analysis and evaluation	Judges the reliability of data and information using pre-defined techniques and/or criteria.	Analyses a range of information, comparing alternative methods and techniques. Selects appropriate techniques/criteria for evaluation and discriminates between the relative relevance and significance of data/evidence collected.	Analyses new, novel and/or abstract data using an appropriate range of established subject-specific techniques. Judges the reliability, validity and significance of evidence to support conclusions and/or recommendations. Suggests reasons for contradictory data/results.
Performance and practice			
Adaptation to practice	Locates own role in relation to specified and externally defined parameters.	Identifies external expectations and adapts own performance accordingly.	Locates own role within poorly defined and/or flexible contexts requiring a level of autonomy.
Performance	Undertakes performance tasks that may be complex and non-routine, engaging in self-reflection.	Undertakes complex and non-routine performance tasks. Analyses performance of self and others and suggests improvements.	Seeks and applies new techniques and processes to own performance and identifies how these might be evaluated.
Team and organisational working	Works effectively with others and recognises the factors that affect team performance.	Interacts effectively within a team, giving and receiving information and ideas and modifying responses where appropriate. Recognises and ameliorates situations likely to lead to conflict.	Works effectively within a team, supports or is proactive in leadership, negotiates in a professional context and manages conflict. Proactively seeks to resolve conflict.
Ethical awareness and application	Demonstrates awareness of ethical issues and is able to discuss these in relation to personal beliefs and values.	Is aware of personal responsibility and professional codes of conduct.	Is aware of personal responsibility and professional codes of conduct and incorporates this into their practice.

Personal enabling skills

	Level 4	Level 5	Level 6
Personal evaluation and development	Is aware of own capabilities in key areas and engages in development activity through guided self-direction.	Assesses own capabilities using justifiable criteria set by self and others taking the wider needs of the context into account. Uses feedback to adapt own actions to reach a desired aim and reviews impact.	Takes responsibility for own learning and development using reflection and feedback to analyse own capabilities, appraises alternatives and plans and implements actions.
Interpersonal and communication skills	Uses interpersonal and communication skills to clarify tasks and identify and rectify issues in a range of contexts.	Adapts interpersonal and communication skills to a range of situations, audiences and degrees of complexity.	Sets criteria for, and is effective in, professional and interpersonal communication in a wide range of situations.

References

Airey, J. 2012. The roller coaster of life as a student nurse. *British Journal of Nursing*. 21(19): 1169–1170.

Bagnardi, M. 2014. A national study on preparedness of new registered nurse graduates. *I-Manager's Journal on Nursing*. 4(2): 16–20.

Bailey, M. and D. Tuohy. 2009. Student nurses' experiences of using a learning contract as a method of assessment. *Nurse Education Today*. 29(7): 758–762.

Ballantyne, H. 2016. Developing nursing care plans. *Nursing Standard*. 30(26): 51–57.

Barksby, J. 2014. Service users' perceptions of student nurses. *Nursing Times*. 110(19): 23–25.

Brown, K. 2013. Community placements for nursing students. *Primary Healthcare*. 23(6): 28–30

Bryant, R. 2005. *Global Nursing Review Initiative Issue 1: Regulation, Roles and Competency Development*. Geneva: International Council of Nurses.

Buerhaus, P., D. Auerbach and D. Staiger. 2016. Recent changes in the number of nurses graduating from undergraduate and graduate programmes. *Nursing Economics*. 34(1): 46–48.

Bull, R. et al. 2015. Supporting graduate nurse transition: collaboration between practice and university. *The Journal of Continuing Education in Nursing*. 46(9): 409–415.

Carey, M., B. Kent and J. Latour. 2016. The role of peer-assisted learning in enhancing the learning of undergraduate nursing students in clinical practice: a qualitative systematic review protocol. *Joanna Briggs Institute (JBI) Database of Systematic Reviews and Implementation Reports*. 117–123.

Clark, L., D. Casey and S. Morris. 2015. The value of Masters degrees for registered nurses. *British Journal of Nursing*. 24(6): 328–334.

Dahlke, S., M. O'Connor, T. Hannesson and K. Cheetham. 2016. Understanding clinical nursing education: an exploratory study. *Nurse Education in Practice*. 17: 145–152.

Davenport, M., A. Ooms and D. Marks-Maran. 2016. Learning about population health through a community practice learning project: an evaluation study. *Nurse Education in Practice*. 17: 43–51.

Directive 2005/36/EC of the European Parliament and of the Council of 7 September 2005 on the recognition of professional qualifications. *Official Journal of the European Union*. L 255: 22–142.

Duffy, K. 1994. *Failing Students Report*. London: Nursing and Midwifery Council.

Esmaeili, M., M. Cheraghi, M. Salsali and S. Ghiyasvandian. 2014. Nursing students' expectations regarding effective clinical education: a qualitative study: clinical education. *International Journal of Nursing Practice* 20(5): 460–467.

Etheridge, S. 2007. Learning to think like a nurse: stories from new nurse graduates. *The Journal of Continuing Education in Nursing.* 38(1): 24–30

Falk, K. et al. 2016. When practice precedes theory – a mixed methods evaluation of students' learning experiences in an undergraduate study program in nursing. *Nurse Education in Practice.* 16(1): 14–19.

Fleming, N. 2001. *Teaching and Learning Styles: VARK Strategies.* London: Fleming Publications.

Fleming, S. 2011. Undergraduate nursing students' learning styles: a longitudinal study. *Nurse Education Today.* 31(5): 444–449.

Flott, E. and L. Linden. 2016. The clinical learning environment in nursing education: a concept analysis. *Journal of Advanced Nursing.* 72(3): 501–513.

Fotheringham, D. and D. Lamont. 2015. Linking theory to practice in introductory practice learning experiences. *Nurse Education in Practice.* 15(2): 97–102.

Gibbs, G. 1988. *Learning by Doing: A Guide to Teaching and Learning Methods.* Oxford: Oxford Polytechnic.

Gordon, M. et al. 2012. Non-technical skills training to enhance patient safety: a systematic review. *Medical Education.* 46: 1042–1054.

Hart, A. and B. Heaver. 2013. Evaluating resilience-based programs for schools using a systematic consultative review. *Journal of Child and Youth Development.* 1(1): 27–53.

Henderson, A. and M. Cooke. 2012. Nursing students' perceptions of learning in practice environments: a review. *Nurse Education Today.* 32(3): 299–302.

Honey, P. and A. Mumford. 2006. *Learning Styles Questionnaire 2006: 80 Item Version.* London: Peter Honey Publications.

Howlin, F. and P. Halligan. 2014. Development and implementation of a clinical needs assessment to support nursing and midwifery students with a disability in clinical practice: Part 1. *Nurse Education in Practice.* 14(5): 557–564.

Ironside, P., A. McNelis and P. Ebright. 2014. Clinical education in nursing: Rethinking learning in practice settings. *Nursing Outlook.* 62(3): 185–191.

Johns, C. 2013. *Becoming a Reflective Practitioner,* 4th ed. New Jersey: Wiley Blackwell.

Knowles, M. E. Holton III and R. Swanson. 2012. *The Adult Learner,* 6th ed. Abingdon: Routledge.

Kolb, D. 2015. *Experiential Learning: Experience as the Source of Learning and Development,* 2nd ed. New Jersey: Pearson Education.

Krathwohl, D., P. Airasian and L. Anderson. 2013. *A Taxonomy for Learning, Teaching, and Assessing: A Revision of Bloom's Taxonomy of Educational Objectives, Abridged Edition.* Harlow: Pearson Education Limited.

Krol, M. et al. 2016. Enhancing student nurse learning through participation in a community based educational program for children and families. *Journal of Community Health Nursing.* 33(3): 139–144.

Lee, R. and J. Fawcett. 2013. The influence of the metaparadigm of nursing on professional identity development among RN-BSN students. *Nursing Science Quarterly.* 26(1): 96–98.

Matthias, A. 2015. Making the case for differentiation of registered nurse practice: historical perspectives meet contemporary efforts. *Journal of Nursing Education and Practice*. 5(4): 108–114.

Merrell, J. and G. Olumide. 2014. 'Work in progress': nurse educators' views on preparing pre-registration nursing students in Wales for practice in multi-ethnic environments. *Journal of Research in Nursing*. 19(6): 490–501.

Müller, F. and J. Louw. 2004. Learning environment, motivation and interest: perspectives on self-determination theory. *South African Journal of Psychology*. 34(2): 169–190.

Muls, A. et al. 2015. Influencing organisational culture: a leadership challenge. *British Journal of Nursing*. 24(12): 633–638.

Nadelson, S. 2014. Online resources: fostering students evidence-based practice learning through group critical appraisals: teaching EBP column. *Worldviews on Evidence-Based Nursing*. 11(2): 143–144.

Nelwati, L. and V. Plummer. 2013. Indonesian student nurses' perceptions of stress in clinical learning: a phenomenological study. *Journal of Nursing Education and Practice*. 3(5): 56–65.

NMC (Nursing and Midwifery Council). 2008. *Standards to Support Learning and Assessment in Practice*. London: NMC.

NMC (Nursing and Midwifery Council). 2010. *Standards for Pre-registration Nursing Education*. London: NMC.

NMC (Nursing and Midwifery Council). 2015. *The Code: Professional Standards of Practice and Behaviour for Nurses and Midwives*. London: NMC

NMC (Nursing and Midwifery Council). 2016. *Quality Assurance Framework*. London: NMC.

Purling, A. and L. King. 2012. A literature review: graduate nurses' preparedness for recognising and responding to the deteriorating patient. *Journal of Clinical Nursing*. 21(23–24): 3451–3465.

Ranjbar. H. 2016. Stress management: an ignored challenge in clinical nursing education. *Nurse Education Today*. 36: 10.

Royal College of Nursing [RCN]. 2010. *The Principles of Accountability and Delegation for Nurses, Students, Health Care Assistants and Assistant Practitioners*. London: RCN.

Schwarz, D. 2016. *How to Success in College and Beyond: The Art of Learning*. Chichester: Wiley-Blackwell.

Skills for Care. 2015. *Impact of Working Longer Hours on Quality of Care*. Leeds: Skills for Care.

Smoker, A. 2010. Is it all just academic? *Dermatological Nursing*. 9(2): 7–8.

Stacey, G., K. Pollock and P. Crawford. 2015. A case study exploring the experience of graduate entry nursing students when learning in practice. *Journal of Advanced Nursing*. 71(9): 2084–2095.

Tonks, J., N. Fawcett and S. Rhynas. 2014. Re-finding the 'human side' of human factors in nursing: helping student nurses to combine person-centred care with the rigours of patient safety. *Nurse Education Today*. 32: 1238–1241.

Warfield, C. and K. Manley. 1990. Developing a new philosophy in the NDU. *Nursing Standard*. 4(41): 27–30.

Watt, E. and E. Pascoe. 2013. An exploration of graduate nurses' perceptions of their preparedness for practice after undertaking the final year of their bachelor nursing degree. *International Journal of Nursing Practice*. 19(1): 23–30.

WHO (World Health Organization). 2010. *Strategic Directions for Strengthening Nursing and Midwifery Services 2011–2015*. Geneva: WHO.

WHO (World Health Organization). 2015. *Options Analysis Report on Strategic Directions for Nursing and Midwifery Services 2016–2020*. Geneva: WHO.

Willis, G. 2015. *Raising the Bar. Shape of Caring: A Review of the Future Education and Training of Registered Nurses and Care Assistants*. London: Health Education England.

Index

Lightning Source UK Ltd.
Milton Keynes UK
UKOW06f1436271217

314798UK00009B/187/P